Invincible
not Invisible

CHANGE YOUR MINDSET
AND YOUR BODY IN
90 DAYS

Synergy Publishing
Newberry, FL 32669
publishwithsynergy.com

Invincible Not Invisible
Change Your Mindset And Your Body In 90 Days
By Fiona Lambert

Printed in the United Kingdom.

Library of Congress Catalog Card Number: 2024930609

International Standard Book Number: 978-0-912106-98-4

Interior Layout and Cover Design:
Cris Convery | hello@crisconvery.com

Commissioning Editor:
Carolyn Andrews | carolyn@publishwithsynergy.com

Disclaimer:
Before beginning any exercise program, please consult with your physician or healthcare provider. The information provided in this book is intended for general guidance and educational purposes only. The exercises and activities outlined in this book may not be suitable for everyone. It is important to listen to your body, make modifications as needed, and stop any activity that causes discomfort or pain. By engaging in the exercises in this book, you acknowledge that you are doing so at your own risk. The author and publisher of this book are not responsible for any injuries or health issues that may result from following the exercises provided.

Invincible
not
Invisible

**CHANGE YOUR MINDSET
AND YOUR BODY IN
90 DAYS**

FIONA LAMBERT

S
Synergy
PUBLISHING

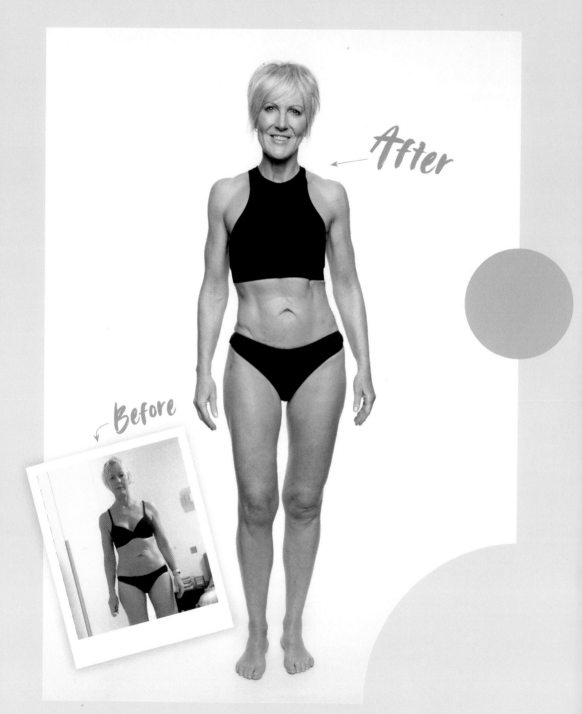

After

Before

To succeed, you need to make brave choices, try new things and squeeze out every last drop of drive and resilience.

CONTENTS

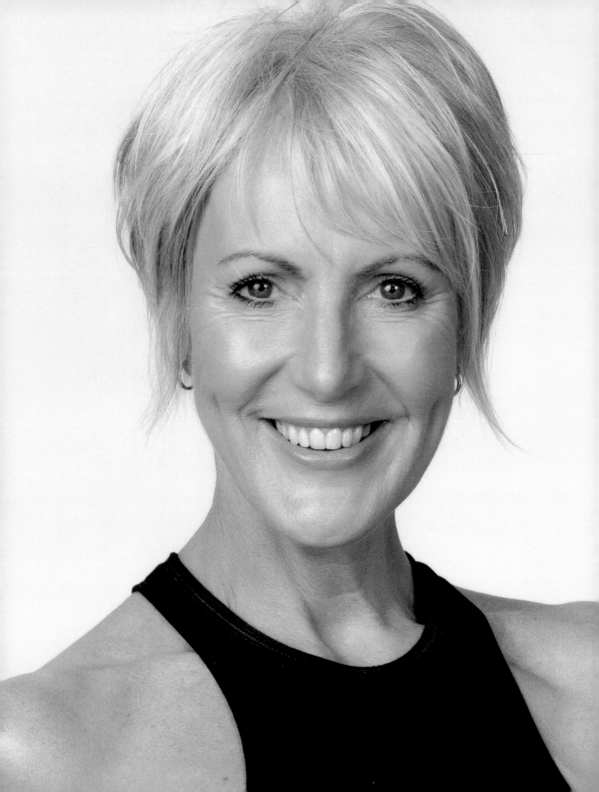

CHAPTER 1

A LITTLE BIT ABOUT ME

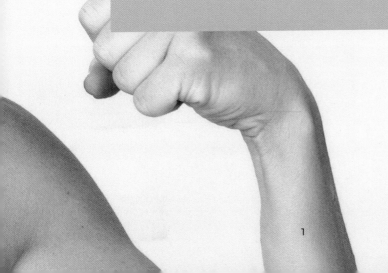

Well, this is a big surprise!

I never expected after a 35-year career in the fashion industry to be talking to you about a fitness goal I set myself at the age of 60 and encouraging you to do the same, whatever your age. But then isn't life sometimes more interesting when the unexpected happens? Especially when this turns out to be one of the greatest things that's ever happened to you!

With a desire to get to my fittest at 60, I used methods and psychology attained from my years in business, creating successful strategies to transform brands, that I knew would work for me. I achieved so much in 90 days that it ended up being covered by *The Times* in their health section and it went viral. It led to so many requests for advice and help, it spurred me to write this book, on how to feel Invincible not Invisible.

I was quite academic at school, but knew at age 11 that I wanted to go into fashion. My mother was a seamstress and so was my grandmother. My great grandfather was a master tailor. I grew up with design, fabric, the hum of the sewing machine and beautiful clothes all around me. I remember kneeling on the floor with my mum wearing a dress she had made and pinning the hem for her. I loved it.

Soon I developed a focused plan to get into the industry as a designer and this led me to work with great businesses and some incredible leaders throughout my career.

I am delighted with what I have achieved and learned during my years in the business. Many of these experiences have shaped who I am and how I think today.

At Next, I was fortunate enough to work in my first role with George Davies, the company founder. I started as a designer and pattern cutter, skills I can still turn my hand to. It was a very small business back then compared to now, and even in my junior position I had a lot of time with George. As the man behind Next, George and Per Una, he is one of the most successful and entrepreneurial fashion retailers around.

The pace, passion and absolute focus on both product and customer at Next thrilled me and I progressed fast, revelling in the challenge. I was the buyer and designer behind all of the dresses and blouses as we launched the first Next Directory.

George had a way of working that I have always tried to emulate. I always noticed how he treated people. Whether it was me as a trainee designer and pattern cutter or a Saturday store assistant right through to the directors of the business, George was interested in you and he always made you feel special. This meant he expected the same high standards and work ethic from you as he did himself. I believe it is a measure of a person that they treat everyone the same, irrespective of position.

After 4 years, George left Next in a boardroom upset. As he had already had such an impact on me, I wrote to him to say how much I appreciated all I had learnt from him and that if he set up anything else, I would love to work for him again. Little did I know what a big impact that one letter would have on the next stage of my career. About six months later, I got a call from George to say that he would like me to join him as a partner in a new business, The George Davies Partnership. He had a new proposition, but couldn't say who it was for or what it would be. It all sounded very mysterious and a little scary. It was a risk to leave an established company as a young buyer to join a start-up, but I believed in George and his vision and couldn't resist the opportunity to build something from scratch.

The project turned out to be the launch of George at Asda. Hard to believe now with nearly all supermarkets having a clothing range, but the idea was revolutionary at the time. We had a tiny start up team of seventeen people in total and we all rolled our sleeves up and worked long hours to launch a new brand in just 9 months. As it was such a small team, I was able to employ both my design and buying skills. Soon I progressed to managerial roles and began to develop an understanding of the financial and planning side of the business. George's drive and innovative thinking have always influenced how I work. He told me "There is no such thing as can't" and I will always try my utmost now to find a solution using connections, resourcefulness, knowledge and creativity. I often use the expression "Be more water". Water will always find a path to its destination by slowly and consistently wearing away a course in the rock. If not, it will find a way to flow around the rock. What it doesn't do is throw its hands up in the air and say I can't get to my goal! I hope you will use the phrase now. Of course, there will always be the odd thing that really can't be achieved, but I know how to find a great alternative. Refusing to accept the status quo and setting ambitious goals for myself are traits that have stuck with me from my time with George.

I worked with George for the next 10 years, during which period I had two children, now 31 and 28. It was during this time that I learnt how to juggle being a mum with a full-time job. I am often asked the best way to do this and my answer is that there is no one right way. It has to be something that works for you both personally and financially. What I did learn was how little time I had to focus on me and I became incredibly efficient in squeezing in some exercise and maintaining a family life, all of which continue to help me now.

Something else I am proud of is pioneering the use of computer aided design (CAD) in the business, if you are under 50 this will sound crazy, but we did all design, textiles and garments by hand prior to this. I was and continue to be interested in the impact of new technology on retail. I am now learning more and more about technology in relation to my health and fitness journey.

By the late '90s I had become the Design Director of George. It was at this time that I was approached to return to Next as their Womenswear Product Director. I was hugely loyal to both George the man and George the brand, but the direction was changing under new ownership (Asda had been purchased by Walmart). The autonomy and passion for product was being waylaid by a desire for lower prices.

I decided it was time to take on another new challenge, a more important role in a more corporate environment with Next. The brand was doing well but there were opportunities to push the design forward and grow the customer base. I was getting out of my comfort zone again!

I stayed at Next for the following 6 years, working closely with Simon Wolfson, who is still the brand's incredibly successful CEO. My big lesson from working at Next was how the use of data, analytics and meticulous planning, together with design, intuition and innovation, makes for an ideal business combination. In a situation where my part to play was complemented by logistics, operation and finance directors, I had to know the facts and data to back up my creative skills.

It takes both ability and courage to confidently book orders costing millions of pounds! The fact is that a fashion brand that doesn't take any risks will stagnate and, ultimately, die. I learned to back my own convictions and began to paraphrase a line from Simon; that I would rather rein in a stallion than drag a donkey, (teams who have worked with me will laugh as they still quote me now). The idea here is that it's better to have a go at something and maybe make the odd mistake than never to try anything at all. If you set yourself up as best as possible for success and build on wins, you gain forward momentum. This all round, holistic approach is what it takes to deliver a successful collection and achieve brand transformation. I will spend more time later sharing how this can help make a successful transformation for you, too.

· · · · ·

"If you set yourself up as best as possible for success and build on wins, you gain forward momentum."

· · · · ·

After six years, I was approached to re-join George to help restore some of the vision and purpose that had been lost in the intervening years under new leadership.

A radical reinvention was required and I believed that I was the woman for the job.

It was the biggest step in my career so far. Until then, my job was to deliver someone else's vision and plan. This move brought plenty of responsibility with £1.6bn in sales

and hundreds of people's jobs relying on me to make the right moves. With a deep breath, I took the role. This meant I had to believe in myself, silencing any inner critic with a focus on all I had accomplished to date.

I am making this sound like it was easy, but I know well how self-doubt can creep in. I have developed many techniques to help manage imposter syndrome and turn my inner critic into a positive belief system. I will also be sharing these techniques as I believe they are a key part of changing your lifestyle.

This new role meant not only transforming the brand with a fresh sense of purpose and vision, but it also required extensive planning and preparation that would enable a huge team to function at the highest possible level.

I knew that it would not be an overnight transformation, as the lead-times for new ranges from scratch, plus a new brand identity, store design and marketing plan would all take 12–18 months to deliver. Patience and perseverance would be required by all. These will be core tenets to remember as we move deeper into our own transformations. Lots of tips to come on this!

During my career I have been fortunate to witness several inspiring people speak. I particularly remember a couple of individuals who influenced me. One said, "If you are in a position of power and influence in a company, it is your duty to do good".

The second said "Life's three stages are about earning, learning and giving". Both resonated with me and I took the advice on board as I moved into more senior roles where I was able make important decisions.

Whilst at George, Graduate Fashion week was set up to support young fashion and knitwear graduates in gaining exposure for their ranges with exhibitions and catwalk shows across London. Things went well until one year the initiative lost its title sponsor at the 11th hour. I had been a judge for the awards for some years and was able to convince the business just how important their support was in keeping the event alive. In my view, these designers were the future lifeblood of the industry.

The business went on to sponsor the awards for another 5 years. This meant that the George brand was not seen solely as a place for cheap clothing (as it had started to become over the years), but was seen as a positive force on the wider industry. This just goes to show that it is never too late to change!

During my time at George, we achieved many other firsts, including selling the winning graduates' collections and holding the first childrenswear catwalk show. We also held workshops at school level to help younger children understand how they could pursue a career in fashion. I have mentored and coached many young designers and buyers and love to watch people blossom. This love of helping others be the best they can is a key reason I decided to write this book.

I have always had an interest in what makes people tick. I wrote my dissertation on "The Psychology of Fashion". I was fascinated in what people buy, why they buy and why they wear what they wear.

To develop great fashion and solutions for customers, you have to decide what they want before they do! Understanding this meant that I always listened to people in order to gain a deep understanding of their needs.

I was surprised and delighted by how many lovely people contacted me when my 60th birthday story hit the press. There have been lots of messages from women who feel they have left it too late or who have lost confidence in their ability to change. For me, it seemed there was a void of inspiration and information on ways to improve your fitness levels in a relatable way, especially as women hit perimenopause.

Throughout my career I have learnt valuable lessons in resilience, life-coaching, planning and psychology. Having worked for brands including George, Next, Dunelm and most recently Jaeger, my job has required huge amounts of energy, commitment and passion, none of which I have lost an ounce of.

When I stopped full time work at the end of December 2022 in order to start consulting, it meant I could invest time in myself for the future.

I set about transforming myself, knowing that I could harness the same skills in order to be the best version of myself. I recognise that mindset plays a huge part in our attitude towards exercise and improving fitness levels.

I was never sporty at school. In fact, I actively avoided sports day to the extent of feigning sickness or tummy aches. I started to enjoy table tennis and badminton when I was about 16 years old. This was the first time that I realised you need to enjoy the physical activity you choose to engage in if you're going to stick to it (more on that later). In my 20's and 30's, family and work commitments limited the time I could invest in fitness (and isn't it so much easier
to stay slim when you're younger?).

As my children were growing up, I managed to get to a couple of classes of whatever the latest craze was. I tried brief stints at the gym but like most members never really got value out of them. I certainly had no love or obsession with keeping fit.

Only in later life, as my children have grown-up and left home, have I realised the benefits of being in the best shape possible. I have discovered the glow of endorphins, the body's natural pain killer that is released after a challenging workout and which makes you feel less stressed, (they are also released with laughter and making love, but let's focus on exercise!). I have realised how keeping fit and toned boosts confidence and fosters a more positive attitude to go out and face the world. Truly, it is the kindest gift you can give yourself.

During the Covid pandemic I found myself without a job after the start-up brand I was part of lost its funding. In lockdown I did two things that, unbeknownst to me, probably set me on this journey.

Firstly, I had more time to invest in my health and fitness. Due to being unable to leave the house, I explored lots of ways to keep fit at home, from tap dancing to creating my own boot camp in the garden with equipment I found around the house. I shared my fitness ideas on social media to keep friends and family entertained and soon found that these were motivating others, which in turn motivated me further.

- - - - -

During the Covid pandemic I found myself without a job after the start-up brand I was part of lost its funding. In lockdown I did two things that, unbeknownst to me, probably set me on this journey.

- - - - -

Secondly, having always been keen to help people develop through coaching and mentoring, I decided to study life-coaching. I learnt so much to support my mindset, including how to set goals, manage time and overcome limiting beliefs. I saw that we often impose our own barriers to success and I learnt how to replace these with positive thinking.

The other major event in my life that happened during lockdown was my son's kidney failure. He was diagnosed as a child with a genetic kidney disorder that meant he was a regular visitor to Great Ormond Street Hospital. During his childhood I juggled a director role at Next with managing this condition. We were always told that his one good kidney would fail one day, but had always been led to believe that this would happen when he was in his forties.

At the end of 2019 my son's kidney function began to rapidly decline and despite us moving quickly to find a live donor, it failed before we were able to. He began dialysis treatment at home which kept him alive, but it was a tough time.

Tougher times were to come. As Covid spread, we realised just how vulnerable his condition made him. All ICU beds were being used for Coronavirus patients, meaning all transplants were put on hold. As someone who has always tried to remain positive, I was devastated. Soon after I got the call to say my job was being terminated. On top of all this, my daughter's wedding was cancelled three times.

The combination of these events meant that I had to find deep reserves of positivity. I found that rather than worrying about the end goal, managing each day, week and month until we were given a transplant date became the best option. Eventually, in October 2020, my son's amazing cousin donated a kidney. He has now had a transplant kidney for almost 4 years and this is one of the things that I am most grateful for every single day of my life.

Although this was an incredibly tough time for my family and I, I am nonetheless thrilled that my personal fitness challenge ended up motivating so many people.

In this book, I am going to share with you all of the tips and tricks I learnt along the way, offering as much support and encouragement as I can. But remember, in the end, only you can choose to make the changes and stick with them. There are always going to be reasons to delay the start of your own challenge. It could be time, cost or a lack of self-belief. All I am asking you for is 90 days of commitment. Give me that and I promise that the impact will be life-changing.

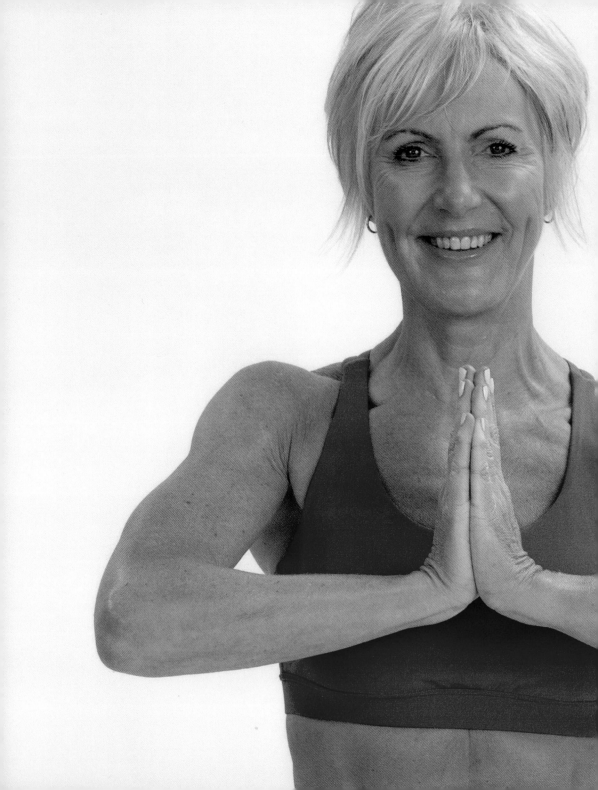

CHAPTER 2

WHY AND HOW
I GOT FIT
AT 60

So, you might ask, why would I decide at 60 to pivot away from a role I have loved and found success in to write a book on fitness goals? Here are the six primary reasons. As you read, start to reflect on what would motivate you.

1. TO PROVE THAT YOU ARE NEVER TOO OLD

I believe there are three different approaches to ageing. First, there are the positive, energetic people who have never made any concessions to age. Many of these people have been fit all their lives and have a lifestyle and mindset that keeps them that way. Looking at them from the outside, it's easy to say they are lucky to have a great metabolism or excellent genes. What you don't see are the positive choices and hard work that comes with taking this path less travelled.

Secondly, there are those who have slowed down, comfortably lapsed into middle-age and begun to make poor choices, notably eating badly and not exercising. For some, this is a happy place to be, and I have no issue with that. They may not be aware of the huge benefits of a healthier lifestyle.

Then there are those whose have had circumstances that have made it difficult to keep on top of their health and well-being, and just don't know how to re-start. If these latter two groups sound like you, I hope you will feel in control again after reading this book.

I'm currently the fittest and leanest I have ever been. Not in spite of being 60, but because I am 60 and want to celebrate this marvellous body machine we have been given. Contrary to what many think, it's not all about genes or working ridiculously hard, but rather altering your lifestyle in a way that feels sustainable. Eating consciously and exercising on a consistent basis is everything. I will share with you all the tips I learned. If I can get into great shape, anyone can. And if I can inspire just one person to choose a healthier lifestyle, then it's all been worth it.

2. TO WORRY LESS AND LIVE MORE

As a painfully shy child, I spent far too long worrying about what people thought of me. I admit, the same goes for my adult years too. What do I wish I could tell my 20-year-old self, even the 40-year-old? Comparison really is the thief of joy. Physically I wanted bigger boobs, thinner thighs, thicker hair, nicer teeth.

At work, I compared myself to my bosses (mostly men) who had completely different skill sets to me and I saw this as a barrier to success. The joy of realising that being the unique, wonderful, incomparable, best version of myself is what I wish I'd known earlier. I want everyone who reads this to feel that joy.

The years I spent working in fashion, developing ranges that have clothed millions of women, their families and their homes, have taught me that how you look has the power to transform your outlook for the day. I love styling and have collected a wardrobe of items I have accumulated over the years. I want to continue wearing the gorgeous things I bought in my twenties and thirties, alongside short skirts and strapless tops that are deemed inappropriate for a woman my age.

It's easy to overthink what to wear, but for me, it's all about having fun, being creative and enjoying fashion. I know though, that if something feels a bit tight and there is a nagging voice at the back of my mind, it's best to take it off. Only when I feel truly comfortable do I most enjoy the friends I'm with or the environment I'm in. Then, I can feel fabulous!

3. TO SHOW YOU ALWAYS HAVE ENOUGH TIME

I remember having a conversation with my boss at the time, about ten years ago now. He was an avid cyclist and managed to pull off 20-mile rides mid-week. What was his secret? Choice. Everything for him was a choice. He wanted to keep fit and loved cycling.

The only way to fit it into working hours was to set his alarm 45 minutes earlier for a 6am wake-up. I remember thinking: 'No way, would you catch me doing that'. But in hindsight something must have resonated because I've since found myself replicating similar trade-offs. However demanding and full-time a role may be, there is always a way to find time to keep fit.

When you have small children, it's tougher to make time for yourself. My children left for university several years ago, so all the 'I don't have the time' excuses are out of the window now. These are choices I make every day. Some of them are big, some small, but they all add up in the end.

Here are several examples:

- Wearing a smart device that prompts me to move every hour and reminds me of my target.

- Walking 10k steps a day.

- Exercising before breakfast. This means I have completed my main fitness regime for the day and makes me feel more energised. Having started the day well, I am already on a roll so less likely to be led astray by temptation.

- Choosing an app which showed me that with ten to fifteen minutes of HIIT training a day (High Intensity Interval Training), I can burn 250 calories. Anyone can find 10 minutes to do this instead of 10 minutes of scrolling on social media.

- Cooking with fresh ingredients. It takes more time than a takeaway or ready meal, but it tastes better and if you make the right choices, it's also healthier.

- Eating slowly and appreciating my meals. This means sitting at a table without a phone or the TV. I look forward to sharing some fast and easy recipes later!

4. TO NOT TAKE MY HEALTH FOR GRANTED.

As I mentioned, my son has had a kidney disorder since childhood. He suffered kidney failure and dialysis in 2020, just as transplants ground to a halt due to Covid. I have elderly parents and I am watching my father lose his mobility. Both situations are compelling me to be as healthy as possible.

Whilst I have this marvellous body machine that is fit and healthy, I want to enjoy the outdoors to the full, to go for a walk in all weather and to embrace the challenges and the flood of endorphins that exercise gives us. Endorphins are the body's natural response to the physical demands of exercise. They trigger a positive, euphoric feeling that relaxes the body and makes you feel optimistic.

A healthy body is a healthy mind. I am certain that the work I've put into my body has contributed to the appetite I have for life and, by extension, my career. I never want to look back and feel I didn't live life to the fullest.

5. TO PUSH MYSELF OUT OF MY COMFORT ZONE

Failure is hardwired into our brain to signal disaster from our earliest days of childhood. That's a shame because failure is how we develop. Despite being a reserved child – maybe because of it – I began to push myself out of my comfort zone early in life. I learnt that getting your fingers burnt is no catastrophe but a gentle and often rewarding lesson. The habit stuck. I have always sought ways to push myself to learn and grow in my personal and professional life. Resting on my laurels – or my backside! – is not for me.

I find deadlines a crucial source of motivation. When it comes to fitness, I signed up for the Yorkshire Three Peaks challenge – climbing the three highest mountains in Yorkshire, which required building up to hike 26 miles. I did a 5k run for charity to build up to a half-marathon.

To succeed, you need to make brave choices, try new things and squeeze out every last drop of drive and resilience.

Having worked in senior positions in the fashion retail world, I learnt that in a cutthroat professional and social environment, it's all about staying ahead of the crowd. To succeed, you need to make brave choices, try new things and squeeze out every last drop of drive and resilience. They are the same traits I employ when working with my PT, Joss. He threw down the gauntlet last year, challenging me to get into the best shape of my life for my 60th birthday. He knew it would inspire me, but also that it would inspire others. This made it a challenge but also gave me a sense of purpose. Of course, I couldn't resist.

6. TO BREAKDOWN THE STEREOTYPE THAT AT 60 YOU ARE OVER THE HILL

Unfortunately, ageism is rife.

You see it in the workplace with who gets hired or promoted. In media and marketing where women, in particular, don't seem to be allowed to age. The advertising and recruitment industry treat us like we are invisible. Only 4% of advertising features people over 60, when we are 22% of the population with 27% of the spend. We have the money, the time, the confidence – so why not involve us? We deserve marketing that doesn't make us feel invisible and is as fun, formidable, fantastic, feisty, fearless, foxy and fabulous as we are!

I hear now, "You don't look 60!". I guess this is seen as a compliment but does beg the question: why should it matter?

When I hear this, I want to ask, "What does 60 look like?"

I always avoided saying my age and as I hit my birthday, I couldn't help but wonder why this was. Maybe because of the industry I worked in, which is always about the latest trend or newest technology. Or maybe it was because I thought I would be judged as less relevant.

Either way, being asked if I'm going to retire when I still have a ton of passion and energy was annoying to say the least.

Frustrated at feeling pigeonholed and side-lined, I wanted to stick two fingers up at the people who judge us negatively and to go out fighting the corner of women (and men) like me.

I didn't go into this thinking I was going to be a model or an athlete. I just set a personal challenge to be the best version of myself. Like many, being regularly faced with the polished versions of people's lives on social media, where youth is idolised, it's too easy to compare yourself to all of the pretty young things out there.

I decided that I wanted to make 60 the start of something. Something to celebrate and not hide from. 60 is about liberation, not limitation, and I am ready to fly the flag.

If you have attempted to change your lifestyle before and haven't been able to stick with it, I'm going to ask you to have another go with me. I am going to ask you to step out of your comfort zone and you will see that, one step at a time, even with the odd step backwards, you will achieve your goal.

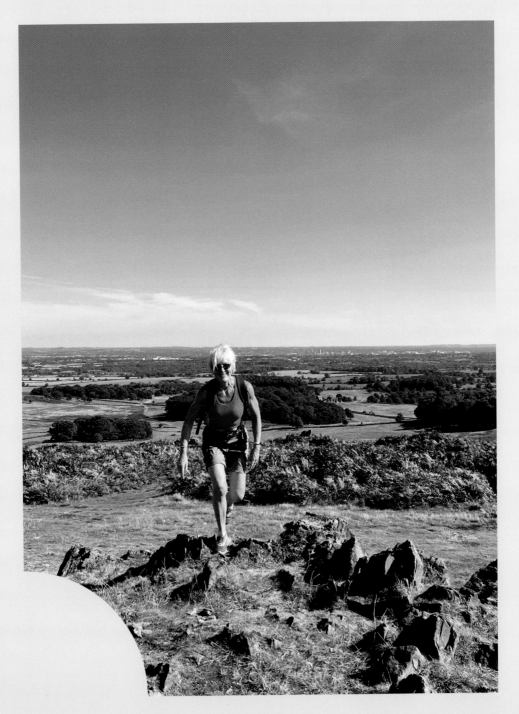

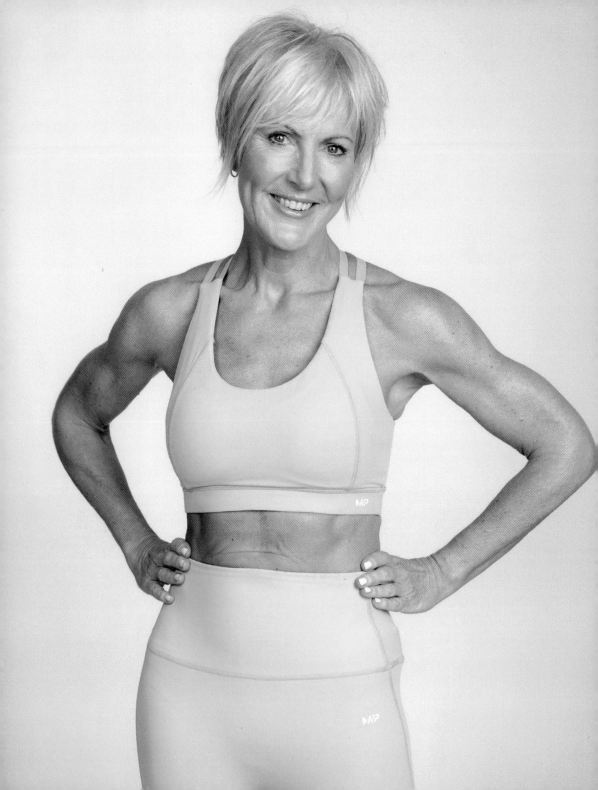

CHAPTER 3

THE 5 WAYS IN 90 DAYS

Have you heard of the 21/90 principle?

It basically states that you can break or create a habit in 21 days. That's not very long, is it? Then, if you can stick at it for 90 days, it becomes your lifestyle and something you can stick with.

So, first things first, we are going to get you in the right mindset to achieve your fitness and health goals. We will then create a plan for the next 90 days of exercise and nutrition. If you can stick with it for 21 days, the rest will get easier and should be really enjoyable, especially as you will start to see results. The exciting thing is that all of this is sustainable. There are lots of 'lose weight quickly' programmes, and lots of celebrity books and DVDs sold, where after a year all of the weight has been regained. This is not a book just about losing weight, it's about being the best version of yourself long term.

Neither is it just a book for 90 days; it's for forever! We are going to embark on an inspiring and motivating adventure to help you achieve not only physical fitness, but also lasting happiness, vitality and fulfilment. Sound good?

HERE ARE THE 5 WAYS.

PURPOSE
PREPARATION
PERSEVERANCE
PEOPLE
POSITIVITY

BEFORE YOU START – ARE YOU REALLY READY?

Take a look at the questions below, I have put where my scores were and knew I had to work on my lower scoring areas (I will confess to not being the most patient of people in the coming chapter on Perseverance). Have a think about the questions and score yourself in the blank grid below mine.

		None 1	Maybe tomorrow 2	Getting there 3	Almost ready 4	Champing at the bit 5
Do you have a really good reason why you want to do this?	**Purpose**					5
How good are you at making a plan and sticking with it?	**Preparation**			3		
How much will power do you have as this won't happen over night?	**Perseverance**		2			
Have you got your cheerleaders lined up?	**People**			3		
Do you believe you can do this?	**Positivity**				4	

YOUR TURN...

Here's your chance to work out how ready you are and if you have the right mindset to make changes and sustain them. We are going to do the same questions when you have read all the tips!

		None 1	Maybe tomorrow 2	Getting there 3	Almost ready 4	Champing at the bit 5
Do you have a really good reason why you want to do this?	**Purpose**					
How good are you at making a plan and sticking with it?	**Preparation**					
How much will-power do you have as this won't happen over night?	**Perseverance**					
Have you got your cheerleaders lined up?	**People**					
Do you believe you can do this?	**Positivity**					

SO ARE
YOU READY?

WHAT'S YOUR SCORE?

1–10
You have probably started so many diets, or joined gyms and have hardly ever gone. By the end of this book you will have so many mental tips and tricks to make this the time you are going to succeed.

11–14
You have probably had some success in achieving what you want but lose momentum and yo-yo. We are going to cut the string on that yo-yo and give you the tools to maintain your success.

15–20
This book is going to just give you the final push to achieve your goals and create a life style that keeps you at peak.

21+
You should be writing this book.

Whatever your score, I promise it will increase when you have read this!

I believe you can and will make a change to your lifestyle in 90 days.

This might be tough love, but are you in or out?

Remember, I'm with you all the way.

Yes? Then let's begin...

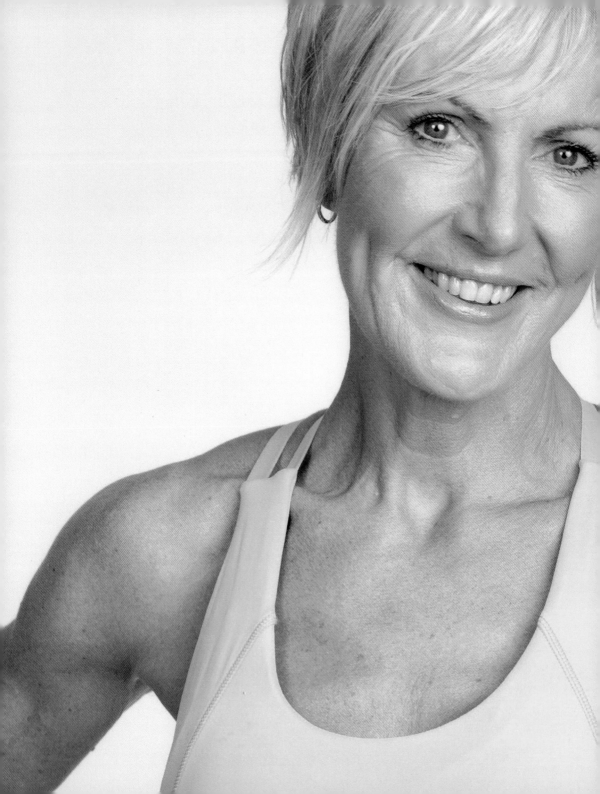

CHAPTER 4

PURPOSE

Now that I have shared the 6 reasons why I wanted to shake things up at 60, it is time to consider your purpose in order to make lasting changes to your lifestyle. Whatever your age this will apply.

Throughout my career, I learnt that the first step to transforming a brand was to understand it's purpose.

To be successful at my job, I have had to understand what is special and unique about each brand. I have learnt not to copy or compare my work with others, but to keep innovating and creating new designs that would continually transform the brand.

If you are feeling unhappy with how you look, it's important to understand that happiness is not just about looking and feeling your best. Often the most beautiful people struggle to feel content. But when you find your passion and purpose, you can create a fulfilling life that is not only more active, but happier.

Your purpose is a personal and unique journey. It's an opportunity to prioritise your own growth, happiness and fulfilment. Embrace this chapter and a new chapter of life with an open heart and a willingness to explore, and you'll likely discover a sense of purpose that brings you joy and satisfaction.

Remember my new purpose is helping others to be the best versions of themselves, so I really want this to work for you!

Before we embark on the next step to firm up your purpose, consider the following:

EMOTIONAL

FUN WITH NEW OR OLD FRIENDS AND YOUR FAMILY

Engaging in group fitness activities or classes can be something you do with friends. It can even provide you with opportunities to make new ones. Exercise with old friends and family will give you experiences to talk about and goals to share. Trying new sports brings different challenges and conversation. (I recently took 3 friends of mine white-water rafting – both great fun and exhilarating!) Following and engaging with instructors or motivational people on social media creates a virtual community of like-minded people, whom you will often get to meet in real life.

FEEL MORE CONFIDENT IN CLOTHES

Whether it's being able to wear old favourites, treat yourself to new things or try stuff on in a changing room without getting stuck inside a top (or is that just me?), you will have less clothing dilemmas when you lose weight. You can walk into a room feeling like a million dollars. I had the fun experience of being asked to model some dresses for an online fashion retailer and thoroughly enjoyed it. I wasn't a rake thin young model, but a confident, healthy 60-year-old. The campaign proved so successful for the brand that I have gone on to do it several more times since.

FEEL LESS STRESSED

Exercise is an effective way to manage stress. We are all spinning plates and multitasking; exercise offers an antidote to the chaos, both physically and mentally.

Physically, it prompts the release of endorphins, the neurochemicals we now know as the "feel-good" hormones. This lifts your mood and fosters a sense of well-being. A surge in endorphins acts as a natural stress reliever, countering the effects of the stress hormones like cortisol, thereby reducing feelings of anxiety and tension. Cortisol also makes you gain weight, promoting the storage of fat, especially around the abdomen. Less stress and less belly fat? That's got to be a win-win.

Regular exercise also stimulates the production of neurotransmitters like dopamine and serotonin, which are important to regulate our mood.

These neurotransmitters help create a sense of calm and contentment, both vital in combatting stress.

On the psychological side, physical activity acts as a distraction from daily irritants. If you ski, you have to focus in order to master the slope. If you are doing a dance class, you focus on the steps. If you are weight training, you are counting the repetitions. Exercise offers a reprieve by shifting focus to the present moment.

* * * * *

Whether it's a brisk walk, a yoga session, or a vigorous workout, exercise promotes mindfulness and relieves stress.

* * * * *

Personally, I find it to be a haven of tranquility in a busy life.

INSPIRE OTHERS

As you prioritise your fitness, glow with newfound confidence and walk with a spring in your step, you will inspire family members and friends to think, "I will have some of that, thank you very much!". It is lovely when you hear that someone's life has improved because they have taken a leaf out of your book.

SENSE OF ACHIEVEMENT

I can't tell you how proud I felt when I saw my before and after photographs! As you look in the mirror, it's too easy to focus on the bits you don't like. But a photo won't lie. I would encourage you to take a before picture, then another 4 weeks later, 8 weeks later and at the end of your 90 days. You will see differences to spur you on. For anyone who has taken up running and seen the change from having to stop at the end of the road to running 5k, the sense of achievement is like a glow inside you.

FINDING THE EXERCISE THAT YOU LOVE

If you find the exercise that you love, whether it's dancing, swimming, hiking, or gardening, it can bring joy and fulfilment to your life like nothing else. You will find yourself evangelical about it, encouraging others to have a go. I personally love high energy, aerobic and anaerobic exercise like Boxercise (great for venting any built-up stress!) and I have become a HIIT advocate.

I will share with you some of the reasons HIIT is particularly effective and the difference between aerobic and anaerobic exercise. Remember to experiment. After all, what is the worst that can happen? You might find more than one exercise you like and be spoilt for choice!

THE PHYSICAL

SLEEP BETTER

Anyone else find they are sleeping worse as hormone levels change? The good news is that there is a clear connection between exercise and improved sleep. Exercise triggers all sorts of physiological responses within the body, releasing endorphins, reducing stress hormones, and modulating body temperature, all of which contribute to a more relaxed state that is more conducive to sleep.

Regular exercise regulates our circadian rhythm, the body's internal clock which governs the sleep-wake cycle. Physical activity helps synchronise this internal clock, telling the body to promote more restful and consistent sleep. The type and timing of exercise can make a difference.

Aerobic exercises, such as jogging, cycling, or swimming, enhance the quality and duration of sleep. This type of exercise elevates the heart rate and body temperature during the workout, promoting deeper sleep as the body cools down post-exercise.

Activities like yoga, tai chi or gentle stretching exercises can have a calming effect on the mind and body, reducing stress and tension.

However, intense physical activity too close to bedtime might elevate adrenaline levels and prevent sleep. So, if you are doing a vigorous workout, do it at least a few hours before bedtime to allow the body to wind down.

LIVE LONGER

I am not going to promise you eternal youth, but if you do exercise regularly, it can help reduce the risk of chronic illnesses such as heart disease, diabetes, osteoporosis, and certain cancers, potentially leading to a longer and healthier life. Want to hang around to enjoy life to the full? Enjoy playing with your children and grandchildren as they grow up? Want to tick all those things off your bucket list you said you'd do when you had more time?

Improving your health now should enable you to do that. At 60 I'd like to think I have a good 30 years ahead of me and I want to be at the healthiest I can to enjoy it.

My bucket list continues to grow all the time. In fact, I may need two buckets!

MAINTAIN/INCREASE MUSCLE MASS

As we age and our hormones change, our muscle mass naturally decreases. Muscles burn more energy than fat, creating a faster metabolic rate. Ever wondered why the food we used to eat happily in our twenties and thirties leads to weight gain in later life? That's why. Strength training exercises can help preserve muscle mass and function.

HEALTHIER HEART AND LUNGS

Want to walk up the stairs without your heart pounding in your chest? As I always take the stairs rather than the lift now, to increase my steps and get some sneaky exercise in, I can vouch that this does improve! Keep building your cardiovascular health to strengthen the heart, improve circulation and reduce the risk of heart disease and stroke as you age.

BETTER BONE HEALTH

Sadly, as we grow older and hormones shift, our bones become more brittle. Weight-bearing exercises like walking and strength training can help increase bone density, strengthen the ligaments and tendons supporting them and reduce the risk of fractures and osteoporosis.

BE HAPPIER WHEN YOU STEP ON THE SCALES

Regular physical activity can help maintain a healthy weight or manage weight loss, which is important for overall health and reducing the risk of obesity-related conditions. It's good not to be too obsessed with scales, however. As we have learned, muscle is denser than fat. I focused on fat burning at the beginning of my transformation, then switched to muscle building. I invested in a set of scales that measures my body fat percentage, so I am not just focused on weight.

BETTER BALANCE AND COORDINATION

This in an investment that will pay off later in life. Balance exercises can help prevent falls and maintain mobility and independence as we age. I have to admit to starting off very wobbly doing a few exercises, but as you strengthen your core muscles, you will notice a difference.

MORE PASSION, MORE ENERGY

Staying active can boost your energy levels and combat tiredness. People often ask where do I get my energy from? The answer is my exercise regime. Exercise sends oxygen and nutrients to your tissues as cardio-vascular health improves. This in turn gives you the energy to handle daily chores, work and other aspects of life. It even boosts confidence and stamina in the bedroom. If you're feeling more confident all round, why not treat yourself to some new lingerie?

MENTAL BENEFITS

WELL-BEING

Oh, the fabulous feeling of endorphins being released as you exercise. These stress-busting hormones can help reduce symptoms of depression and anxiety, improve mood, and boost overall mental well-being.

If you are someone who suffers with loneliness, finding groups to exercise with can bring you in contact with people who are like-minded and reduce those feelings. Group activities can also help you get to a stage where exercise is not a chore, but a joy!

BETTER COGNITIVE FUNCTION

Increased physical activity has been linked to improved cognitive function and a reduced risk of cognitive decline and dementia. Learning new exercises and routines is not only exercising your body, it's exercising your brain too. When I signed up to learn Salsa, having to remember new steps and moves every week was a great way to flex both my body and brain.

On the whole, any exercise that uses hand-eye coordination has been proven to slow down decline in cognitive function.

ADAPTABILITY AND RESILIENCE

If you commit to regular exercise, you will be thrilled as you progress. Yet, it is important that your chosen activity challenges you and keeps pushing you more as you improve. Meeting these obstacles will feel easier because you can look back and see how far you have already come. Your body and your mind will adapt and you will build flexibility and resilience both mentally and physically, making it easier to adapt to life's challenges. I was never into running, but I signed up for a 5k run to raise money for a cancer charity after my grandmother was diagnosed. I could barely run 100m, but I persevered and built up little by little. Soon my body adapted and I went on to run that 5k before setting a target for 10k, knowing that I could do it.

Okay, now I am going to have a stab at some negatives.

Here are some of the cons…

YOUR CLOTHES MAY GET TOO BIG

All those things you've not felt confident enough to wear? They now have your name on them. If you have favourite things, you may have to invest in getting them tailored to fit your new dimensions.

YOU LOSE 15 MINUTES A DAY ON TIKTOK/ INSTAGRAM/FACEBOOK

I mean what will those cute kittens do if you don't watch them? And those ingrown hairs? Maybe they won't be removed if you don't give them your full attention. You will get so much more out of life and the video creators won't miss one less follower.

SOME PEOPLE MAY NOT LIKE THE NEW YOU AS MUCH.

If there are people out there who don't like you fitter, happier and more confident, do you want them in your life anyway? Or for that matter, people who only want to socialise with you if you are eating and consuming large volumes of alcohol?

Embarking on a new lifestyle journey will give you a chance to edit your contact list and invest your time with the wonderful people who are so proud of you and what you have done to improve your life.

Why not try writing your pros and cons? You can always pin them up somewhere or keep the list as screensaver to serve as a reminder.

STILL UNSURE?

One last exercise that could help you find your why is one that is often used in business or engineering. It is the process of asking five whys. This is an activity that encourages you to dig below the surface in order to find your true motivation. It may not take five, it could take seven or even more. It's all about whatever works for you.

Here's me using myself for an example:

WHY DO YOU WANT TO GET FIT?

Because I have my 60th birthday this year and want to be at my fittest.

WHY DO YOU WANT TO BE AT YOUR FITTEST AT 60?

Because I don't want to feel that 60 is the start of getting old.

WHY DO YOU NOT WANT TO GET "OLD"?

Because I want to be healthy and fit enough to continue to enjoy life to the full.

WHY DO YOU THINK YOU NEED TO BE FIT ENJOY LIFE?

Because I see my father struggling with weight and mobility and want to remain active for as long as I can.

WHY DO YOU WANT TO STAY ACTIVE?

I have a third of my life left to live life to the fullest and I want to prove to myself and others that age is no barrier.

WHY DO YOU WANT TO PROVE IT TO OTHERS?

Because I get fed up that society starts to treat us like we are invisible as we age; I want to feel invincible, not invisible!

Has reading the pros and cons helped you define your why?

I am going to ask you to fill in this, I have done an example.

I WANT TO GET FITTER AND HEALTHIER BECAUSE

I want to enjoy an active life to the full. I still have a third of my life to go and a long bucket list to tick off.

I think society treats us like we are invisible after 60 and I want to prove it can be the start rather than the end of leading a fulfilling life.

IT'S GOING TO MAKE ME FEEL

Confident, happy in my own skin and invincible, not invisible

IN 90 DAYS, I AM GOING CELEBRATE BY

Having a photoshoot to celebrate what I have achieved.

Now, your turn to fill in the blanks in the following sentences. They will help you to define your unwavering purpose,

I WANT TO GET FITTER AND HEALTHIER BECAUSE

IT'S GOING TO MAKE ME FEEL

IN 90 DAYS, I AM GOING CELEBRATE BY

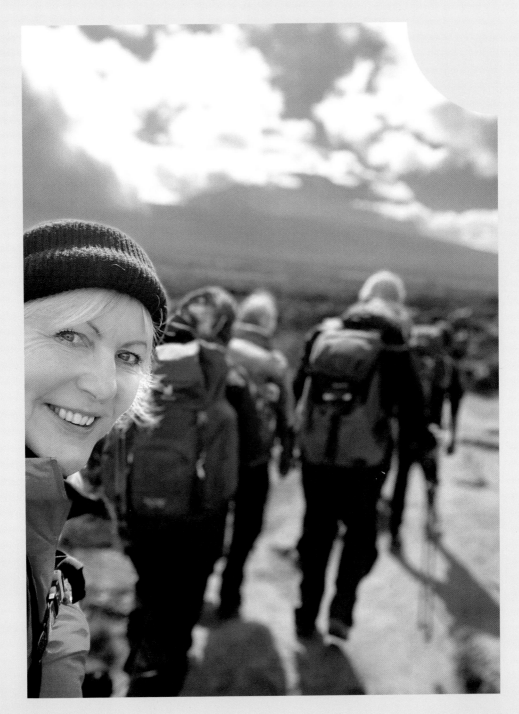

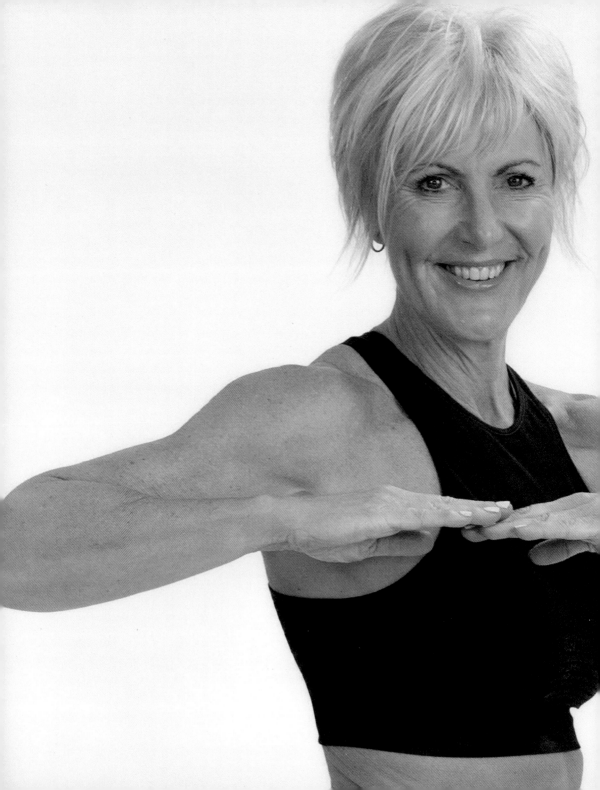

CHAPTER 5

PREPARATION

SETTING YOU UP
FOR SUCCESS

You have taken the first amazing step and found your purpose, using it to set yourself a goal. Let's now make it even more achievable by getting properly prepared.

"Fail to prepare, prepare to fail" as they say. This is your starting point so don't skimp on this stage, take it seriously and your future-self will be extremely grateful that your past-self did such a good job at the beginning by laying some solid foundations.

In the fashion industry we would work to a critical path. This was the length of time it takes to get that beautiful dress you see on a hanger, from design concept to the finished article. This process could take 3 to 9 months and required meticulous planning and lots of moving parts functioning in the correct manner.

The process looked something like this:

Create a mood board of ideas that inspired.

Design the item so that you have an exact picture with which to begin the process. Now the goal is to make this abstract design a reality.

Start sourcing the components that you will need: the fabric, the print design, the buttons and trims, the pattern pieces that magically transform something two dimensional into three.

In order to hit the deadline, you will need to break down the manufacturing process into stages, all of which need to be completed in order for your creation to be ready for purchase.

First, a sample machinist makes a prototype. Tweaks will probably be needed and a second sample will be made. The fabric will then go into production and a print mill will add the colourful design. On delivery of the fabric the manufacturer will cut and sew the dress before it is delivered to the warehouse. A photograph will be taken and uploaded to the website before any orders are picked and delivered by courier. And voila! Your dress arrives like magic!

As shoppers browsing online, we are so used to adding items to our basket at the click of a mouse or the swipe of a finger. The dress of your dreams arrives in the post the next day and we don't consider the nine months of work that went into creating it. We want that dopamine hit now!

I wanted to paint this picture for you as we all want the euphoria of looking and feeling like our vision, but setting yourself up for success requires a clear goal!

So how does this relate to your goal? Let us imagine now that we are designing you. You are the beautiful dress that in three to nine months time will be everything you dreamed of.

To turn this into a plan, we can use SMART.

Have you heard of creating a SMART goal? If you have, feel free to skip this detail, but it is one of the best ways I know to turn a goal, whether it's a business idea, or a personal goal, into a reality.

It stands for:

S – *Specific*
M – *Measurable*
A – *Attainable*
R – *Realistic*
T – *Time-bound*

SPECIFIC:

Write down your goal with as much detail as possible. This turns the goal into a concrete vision. It helps you to articulate and visualise your plan, bringing it to life. We are going to create a mood or vision board which will be the physical embodiment of your purpose.

MEASURABLE:

So how would you like to monitor your progress? I knew that to hit 9st 5lb in 9 weeks from 10st 2lb I would need to lose 1–2lbs per week (if you're a kg person that's approximately 68kg to 60kg losing approximately 1kg per week) Your target may be weight or fitness-based. It's your goal. Whatever it is, it has to be measurable.

ATTAINABLE:

Make sure that your goal is achievable. Nothing is going to de-motivate you more than feeling slightly disappointed every day because your goal was over ambitious. Focus on what you can do and do it.

REALISTIC:

There will be practical requirements or restrictions to accomplishing this goal and you need these to be recognised before commencing.

TIME-BOUND:

This is the deadline by which your goal will be achieved. Setting a time frame stops the end of your goal from drifting continually out of sight. It definitely prevents procrastination. We are going to achieve wonders in 90 days that will change your entire lifestyle! (If you want to set further goals after that, make sure to use the process again).

PLANNING AND PREPARATION

CREATING A VISION BOARD

Visualising success works. Michael Jordan said, "I visualised where I wanted to be, what kind of player I wanted to become. I knew exactly where I wanted to go, and I focused on getting there."

If you can picture yourself in the position you want to be and believe, with positive energy, that you can get there, you are more likely to achieve the outcome you want.

I wanted to reach my 60th birthday and feel fit, confident and at my best. I had a target weight of 9st 5lb (60kg) which was what I weighed on my wedding day. As a treat to myself, I planned a photoshoot at the end that would serve as a celebration of how far I'd come. It was to be a birthday present to myself!

I pulled out the outfits I wanted to wear and collected magazine images that mirrored what I wanted to achieve with regard to lighting and poses. I wanted to be colourful and vibrant, the antithesis

of greying! I found pictures from Women's Health Magazine that showed toned, smiling, fit and confident women. I collected these pictures and created a board that I could refer to in the 11 weeks until my birthday (as it happened the photoshoot was 2 weeks earlier, so I pushed my schedule even harder!). I had my board on my laptop so that whenever I discussed my plans with anyone or contacted a photographer, I could see my goal in physical form.

Some find it more effective to cut out pictures from magazines and create a physical board. However, you do it, make it something you can look at regularly. Pin that board on a wall, or the fridge, or use it as a screen saver.

So over to you.

Think about your goal and the purpose. Find the pictures that embody your vision. Whether its playing with your grandchildren, a holiday, or your very own photoshoot, which I would highly recommend as motivation!

BREAK DOWN THE GOAL INTO (LOW CALORIE) BITE SIZE CHUNKS

Divide your long-term goals into smaller, manageable milestones. This way they don't seem intimidating, impossible, or incomprehensible. As an example, my goal to lose 11lbs in 9 weeks seemed a tough one as I had not been at this weight since before I had children.

When I broke it down, I realised that I needed to lose just 1–2 lbs per week in order to achieve this, which seemed completely doable. As each week passed and new habits formed, I was soon 5lbs down. I knew that I could keep it up. If your goal is to run 5km, break it down into smaller goals.

When I trained to do a half-marathon I gave myself 3 months to train. See the example of my plan below.

WEEKS 1–2	3 miles 2 days per week Sunday 4 miles
WEEKS 2–3	3–4 miles 2 days per week Sunday 5 miles
WEEKS 3–4	3–4 miles 2 days per week Sunday 7 miles
WEEKS 5–6	4 miles 2 days per week Sunday 9 miles
WEEKS 7–8	4–5 miles 2 days per week Sunday 10 miles
WEEKS 9–10	8 miles 2 days per week Sunday 11 miles
WEEK 11	4–5 miles 2 days per week Sunday 12 miles
WEEK 12	3–4 miles 2 days per week Sunday 13.1 miles

Try to apply this level of planning to achieving your goal, it will make the process significantly more manageable.

PLAN YOUR DIARY TO SUCCEED

I am sure that like me you have a diary in which you pencil appointments that help maintain your appearance. Or a work diary where you might schedule training courses to help improve your future career prospects. Would you just decide not to do these because you couldn't quite be bothered?

Well, now you need to create an exercise diary and treat it with just as much importance. View these sessions as equal to having your nails or hair done, in fact afford them even more importance! The healthier, more confident future you, is relying on you. No excuses! Commit one week at a time, make it to 3 weeks (this sets a new habit, remember) and before you know it you will be 90 days in.

REMOVE TEMPTATIONS. REPLACE WITH GOODNESS!

There are lots of tricks to help you replace bad habits with good ones.

Taking away triggers is a good place to start. If you always snack with your coffee, refill your water bottle and take a walk when you would normally reach for a cupcake. If you desire some sort of snack whenever you go to a particular place, try avoiding it for a while (it is a well-known piece of advice to never shop when you're hungry!). It doesn't need to be forever, just until you gain the confidence that comes with lasting change.

It's also worth thinking about other triggers you may have. Is it comfort from food? Numbness from wine? Are you engaging in these behaviours to alleviate stress? Once identified, work out if these triggers can be replaced with healthier ways to achieve a similar feeling.

Habits that are satisfying and relatively simple work best. For example, if you always go to the fridge when you're stressed, try meditative breathing for a while instead of eating and see how you feel. Or count to 100 until the urge passes. All the while, acknowledge that you are making a healthier choice!

If you can't avoid temptation (guilty!), avoid buying the naughty treats and buy healthier ones. I love a pack of flaked salmon or calamari rings and always keep packets in the fridge. You will also find once you've become accustomed to eating differently that you don't crave unhealthy items like you once did. One last tip on this subject: if you make the temptation unattractive (Actor Lesley Ash described squirting washing up liquid onto her children's left over chips to avoid eating them!), it can be resisted quite easily.

REMOVE OBSTACLES

These may be practical or mental. If you can identify them before you start, make strategies to avoid them or pre-plan a solution. It will help. Recognise the situations, emotions, or people that could derail you and trigger those bad habits.

I found it helped during the first couple of weeks to say no to big, boozy social events. This broke the habit of having a glass of wine in my hand. Instead, I planned theatre trips or made an effort to cook special but healthy meals. Have a think about what might get in the way of success and plan out different scenarios to help surmount these obstacles.

One thing that works for me is putting my trainers in a really obvious place near my bed, so that when I wake up in the morning, I can almost trip over them. That way, I am forced to put them on along with my gym kit, rather than my dressing gown.

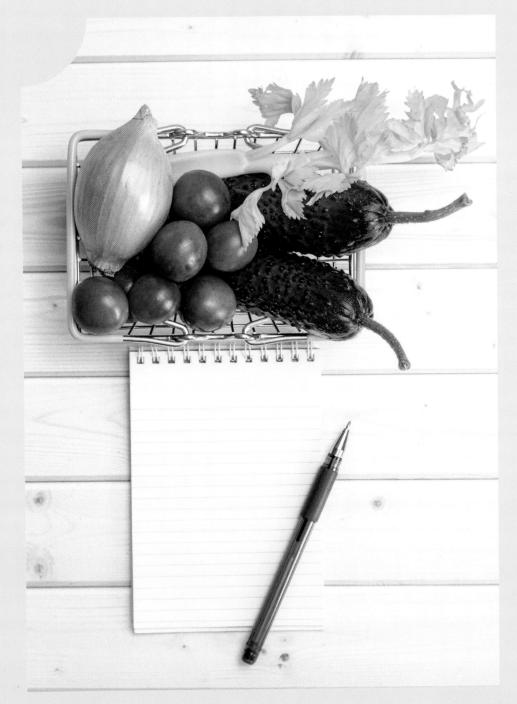

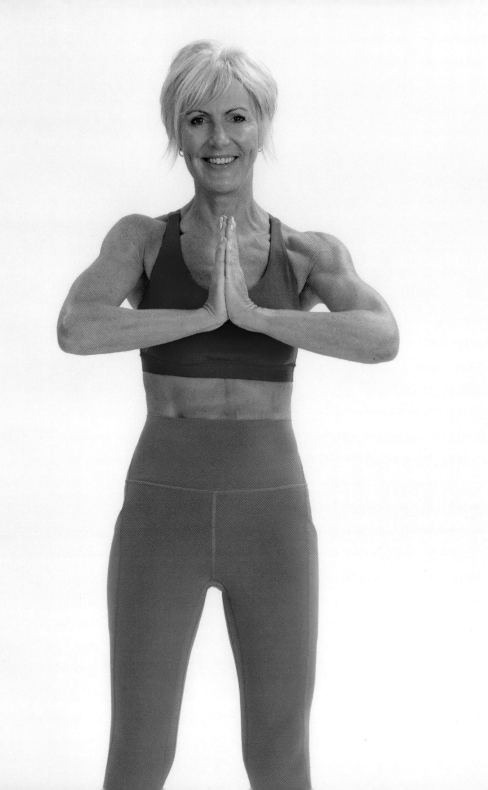

CHAPTER 6

PERSEVERANCE

I am definitely not a very patient person.

It doesn't help that today's world is geared towards instant gratification. Whether that's the latest film streaming on Netflix, ordering a new dress online or awaiting a takeaway from Deliveroo (I think you will be saying goodbye to those for a while, unless it's a healthy grocery shop!).

The most important thing is to remember that this is a lifestyle change, not a quick fix. Impatience for quick results when pursuing personal goals, whether it's in fitness, your career, or any other aspect of life, is something I have had to learn to manage.

While it's natural to want to see rapid progress when you are making changes (and they will feel like sacrifices while you adjust) it's important to manage impatience. In order to avoid regressing, you will need to accept that these are changes you will be making for the long haul.

The reality is that you are going to get bored sometimes. A good exercise programme will by default involve repetition. I am constantly finding ways to make my routines more engaging, whether it's increasing the repetitions to beat my last goal, having new music to work out to or meeting a friend to exercise with.

A healthy diet will have a lot of the same components. I am always on the lookout for new recipes or ways to use ingredients. I also enjoy offering to cook for or with friends in order to share ideas.

The reason I believe so strongly in the 21/90 principle is that, even for an impatient person like me, 3 weeks really isn't a very long time. If you can do 21 days, you will get to 90. Here are some tips that helped me persevere throughout the process.

RECOGNISE THAT THIS IS NOT GOING TO HAPPEN OVERNIGHT

Sadly, there is no Genie with a magic lamp who is going to give you three wishes, of which one of these might be "Let me wake up tomorrow and my goal be achieved!". The reality is that there will be days and weeks where you don't see progress, but stay persistent.

Habits are not broken overnight. Remain committed to the process, even when it feels difficult. Over time, your new, healthier habits will become more and more ingrained. The great news is that the longer you stick to this, the more it becomes a lifestyle.

If you haven't been exercising, the timeline will look something like this.

FIRST 6 WEEKS

This feels like a chore but I will do it as I am going to achieve my goal

6 MONTHS IN

I am enjoying doing this and how it makes me feel

AFTER 1 YEAR

I can't miss my workout / dance class / hike! I love it!

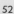

SET REALISTIC EXPECTATIONS

(Remember the R of SMART?) Be realistic about what you can achieve in your time frame. This is especially true if your goal is ambitious or you've not done any exercise for a long time. Meaningful and lasting progress will take time, so get your head in the right place before you start. Understand that progress is rarely linear. If you look at my weight chart it bounces up and down, but what really matters are the weekly results. There will be plateaus and setbacks along the way, but these are all normal parts of the journey.

VIEW YOUR GOAL AS A SET OF STEPS, NOT A LONG JOURNEY

We spent the last chapter planning and preparing to achieve your goal by creating a roadmap with smaller, manageable milestones. It is important to celebrate every bit of progress. Whether it's small daily things like hitting 10,000 steps or saying no to the glass of wine you were offered, or finding at the end of the month that your jeans are too loose. Remember to give yourself a big pat on the back every single day to keep yourself motivated.

CELEBRATE WINS

While we are on celebrating, write down a list of things that are a treat that aren't food or drink related. These can be things that bring you joy and which you look forward to. A long walk with a friend? A new scented candle? A trip to the theatre? For each milestone, write down your treat so that you have a tangible incentive.

My big celebration at the end was my photoshoot and knowing I would feel like a million dollars. I booked and paid for it so it was definitely going to happen.

Write down a list of treats here:

SMALL DAILY TREATS FOR WHEN YOU HIT 10,000 STEPS OR STICK TO YOUR CALORIE GOAL

WEEKLY TREATS FOR WHEN YOU LOSE 1KG

A BIG TREAT FOR MANAGING THAT FIRST 21 DAYS

THE CELEBRATION AT THE END OF 90 DAYS!

ENJOY THE RIDE

Move the focus of your attention from the end result to the process itself. You're learning new things, new recipes, new exercises. You are learning about yourself seeing what works for you. You may be meeting new people or engaging in different conversations from those you would usually have.

Enjoy the journey and find satisfaction in these moments, noting the steps you have taken toward achieving your goals. This is an opportunity for personal growth and self-discovery, as well as a fitter and healthier you. Embrace the learning that comes with it.

STAY CONSISTENT

The good and the bad news is that consistency is key to success. You will be committing to your goals and maintaining a regular routine even when you don't see immediate results. It's often the cumulative effort of lots of small, repetitive programmes and routines that lead to significant change.

OK, you could find this a bit boring to hear, but it works. If you have a wobble such as a long weekend away (as I write this, this is me) where you have maybe eaten or drank too much, don't let this derail you. It's not all ruined. Just start again on the right track.

We are in this for the long game and your new lifestyle is not going to be without the odd day off from your routine, so this is a good lesson to take forward.

LEARN FROM WOBBLES

Having the odd setback is fine. But what if you find you have too many wobbles? In this case, you need to work out what the triggers are. Always want a biscuit when you have a coffee break? Change the process. Top up a water bottle and have an alternative like a packet of really sweet cherry tomatoes on your desk. Always have wine with a meal? Put a large bottle of sparkling water by your wine glass and keep topping up with that. Same friends who always lead you astray?

Try to stay away for a couple of weeks while you make new habits or do something different with them to change the narrative. Book a white-water rafting trip! I did that and it was truly exhilarating.

View setbacks as opportunities to learn and grow.

55

Work out what helps you on your journey and what makes you wobble. Analyse what went wrong, make necessary adjustments and use your newfound knowledge to create a better lifestyle and support network. Remember, it's not about perfection; it's about progress. We all have our moments of indulgence, but that's okay as long as we bounce back stronger.

DEVELOP YOUR PATIENCE

Patience is a virtue. Yes, I have confessed it's not my strongest trait, but you can cultivate patience and improve. Try taking a deep breath, counting to ten or practicing mindfulness when you feel impatient. Remember that patience is a valuable life skill and it can significantly enhance all aspects of your life.

RESEARCH WHAT'S HAPPENING TO YOUR BODY

If you're growing impatient due to a lack of progress, I found that researching the benefits to my health, longevity and hormones really helped me to persevere. You won't look at exercise or a plate of food in the same way. I have been studying personal training as well as learning more about what I have been eating and I will be sharing more of this in the chapters on nutrition and exercise.

ADAPT

Evolution was not survival of the fittest, but survival of the most adaptable (although we should all aim to be both fit and adaptable). Be open to adjusting your approach if it's not yielding results as quickly as you'd like. Sometimes a change in strategy or tactics can lead to faster progress. Some days, if I felt I had plateaued, I fasted until lunchtime.

Fasted exercise seemed to kick start progress both mentally and physically. This worked for me, but it's important to see what works for you. Experiment with when you have your biggest meal of the day, when you exercise and how energetic you feel depending on how much sleep you have. These changes might be all you need.

STOP COMPARING

Avoid comparing your progress and methods to those of others. Everyone's journey to reach their goal is unique. You are finding what exercise you enjoy in order to find a lifestyle that you can maintain. It's not anyone else's life. I am sharing what worked for me. Fasting works for some, keto for others. Try to stay focused on your plan, your routine and your purpose.

TRAIN IN SHORT, SHARP BURSTS

One of the reasons I love HIIT is that it is incredibly effective in a short period of time. When I studied life coaching and had to write assessments for the first time in years without a fixed deadline, I became easily distracted and found that I had a short attention span. I discovered the Pomodoro method which really helped me (I am using it while writing this too!).

POMODORO TECHNIQUE (NAMED AFTER THE TOMATO SHAPED KITCHEN TIMER)

This time management method asks you to alternate pomodoros – focused work sessions – with frequent short breaks to promote sustained concentration and stave off mental fatigue. This is a good technique to turn to if you are easily distracted, have a lot of open-ended work with a distant deadline and would benefit from gamifying your goal setting.

Here's how it works...

- Identify the task
- Set a 25 min timer
- Work on the task until the time is up
- Take a 5 min break
- Every 4 Pomodoro's take a longer 15–30 min break

There are a further 3 rules to make this method work...

- Break down complex projects that require more than 4 Pomodoro's into smaller actionable chunks so you can make clear progress.
- Bundle small tasks together into one session
- Once a Pomodoro is set, focus must not be distracted from that task by email checking, texting or chatting. Any distractions need to be noted down and returned to later.

This technique hinges on the setting of manageable goals in order to prevent procrastination. Momentum breeds momentum. The Pomodoro technique really helps you see what can be achieved in a 25 min segment.

If I know that I can do a 15–20 minute HIIT session, I can also squeeze in a couple of 30 minute walks in the day and make sure that I climb the stairs rather than using a lift or escalator. This way, I am achieving a lot without getting bored or distracted.

AND LASTLY, KEEP GOING BACK TO YOUR PURPOSE

Remember why you set your goals in the first place. Get that vision board out, dig out your why and keep the bigger picture in mind. It will help maintain that all-important long-term perspective.

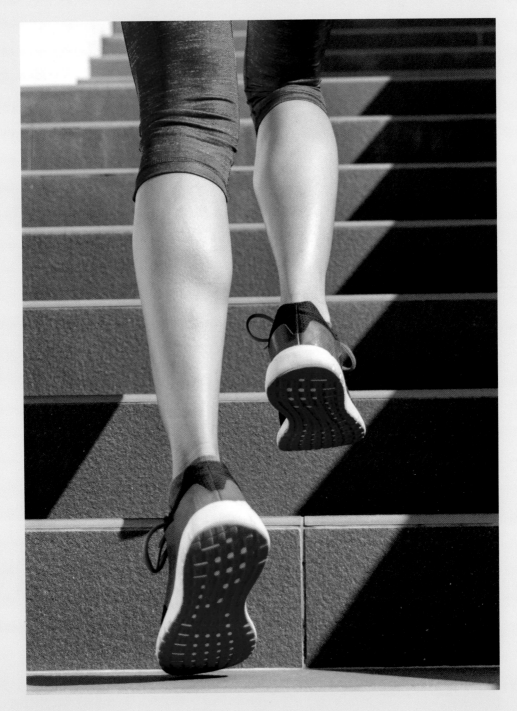

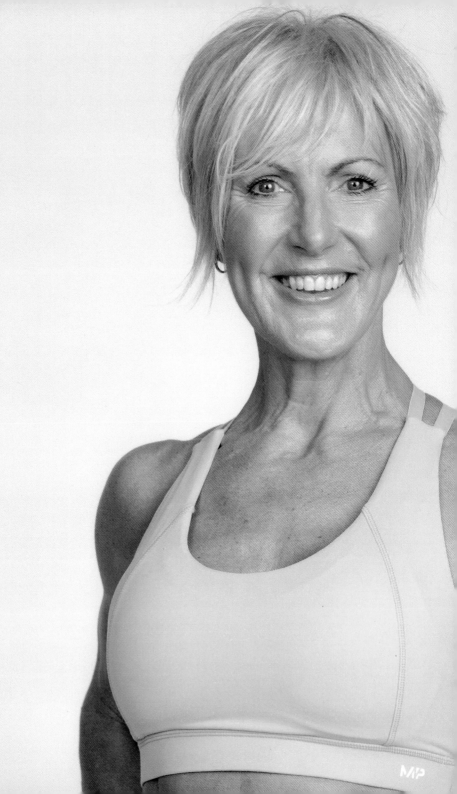

CHAPTER 7

PEOPLE

YOUR SUPPORT NETWORK

There is a well-known quote: "Show me your friends and I will show you your future".

The people around you – who you talk to and who you share with – are going to massively influence your chances of success. By enlisting the support of carefully chosen friends and family and sharing your goal with them, you are multiplying belief in getting and staying where you want to be. By verbalising and sharing your goal with others, you are making it a thing.

I shared my goal to get into the best shape of my life 60, as it was going to mean changes to my diet, social life and exercise routine. I wanted as much support as I could get to bolster my own determination. It's not weak to enjoy support and it's important not to think you have to do everything alone.

FAMILY

You spend lots of time with your family and mine are certainly feeders! I am sure they would say the same of me. I love to cook and entertain. The creative in me enjoys trying, then adapting recipes. I enjoy planning meals and setting a welcoming table. It's one of our ways of showing love.

My dad (86 as I write) was a late starter to cooking but enjoys serving up an old school Sunday roast and traditional puddings like apple crumble, plying us with wine as we eat.

If you are going to adjust your diet to support your goal, you will need to share your goal, but more importantly your "why", with your family.

They will have to understand how important this is to you and be prepared to support you all the way. My dad has now realised that I am not rejecting his cooking (or his love) when I say no to apple crumble because he knows the reasons why.

When I cook at home, I make balanced meals, but my family are used to me turning down potatoes and filling my plate with green vegetables instead.

FRIENDS

Sharing my goal with my friends and making them cheerleaders for me made it all feel real.

Giving up alcohol (especially a glass of white wine) for two months was tough but asking friends to support rather than saying "go on just have one!" really helped.

Again, sharing your purpose is important. You will have some friends who will be super proud of you, even some who may want to join you. If they are good friends, they will check in on your progress. They will be with you, celebrating all the small achievements as you are ticking off the milestones on the way to your bigger goal.

You may also have friends who aren't as supportive. It may be that they have their own issues or that they are short of time or positivity themselves. They may secretly not want you to succeed as its more comfortable for them if you are overeating/drinking and not feeling your best.

Choose which friends you spend lots of time with now and in the future, as they will support your new lifestyle.

FIND AN ACCOUNTABILITY PARTNER

When I shared my goal with my friends, one of them was due to get married 9 months later. She loved what I was doing and set her own goal. We committed to long walks together at weekends. Once you have booked this in your diary, it's a commitment and you won't find any excuses. We shared updates every Sunday on progress, with whoops of encouragement and hugs. Find a friend or family member who can offer support, tips, encouragement and motivation for added accountability.

PERSONAL TRAINER OR FITNESS PROFESSIONAL

If you can afford a PT (new online trainers make it much more affordable), they are another great support mechanism.

My PT, Joss, was not only one of the key drivers for me to get into the best shape of my life at 60, he helped me plan the best exercises to decrease body fat, increase muscle and target my least favourite bits. As he saw me weekly, rather than every day, he could see the progress and offered congratulations and encouragement that kept me motivated and on track. He got me to try new things that pushed me out of my comfort zone and continues to do so. He is thrilled with my achievement as I was a project (albeit a willing one) that he took huge pride in. It was a measure of how good he is at his job.

FIND A SUPPORTIVE COMMUNITY

This can be virtual or physical.

I had no idea when I set out in January 2023 to transform myself that I would post on social media to thousands of people. I am lucky to be part of a community of many fabulous women who motivate, support and joke with one another. I have found an incredible network of like-minded individuals online who share my goals and aspirations as I support and encourage them in theirs. Being part of a community like this grows my passion and reinforces my purpose. I have a real sense of belonging.

Virtual communities on Facebook and Instagram offer websites, exercise programmes, diet tips, shared experiences and before and after pictures that always motivate. The nice ones always reply to questions and comments and other followers offer their support with advice. But if you want real life...

JOIN A CLASS OR LEARN A NEW SPORT

Joining fitness or dance classes is a great way to try different types of exercise, but it also holds you to a commitment of time invested in your goal. I joined a 6-week Salsa dance class for beginners in January. I met new friends who were like-minded and found something recreational to do that wasn't eating and drinking. It was fun, aerobic activity and hey, I learnt basic Salsa, so what's not to love?!

From boxercise to bowling, tennis to trampolining, ping pong to pilates, there will be something out there for you to enjoy alongside others who are investing in their health.

MIX IT UP

It's important to spend time with people of different ages, learning their perspectives, sharing their knowledge and bouncing ideas off each other. At 81 my mum still swims twice a week and walks 10,000 or more steps. She continues to inspire me.

Playing frisbee with my son keeps the big kid in me happy, whilst since lockdown I have talked every week with an elderly gentleman of 87 after Age UK connected us as part of a scheme to battle loneliness. 4 years on we still chat every Sunday. I talk to him about the book and he introduced me to the 369 method of manifestation, which I will share in the next chapter.

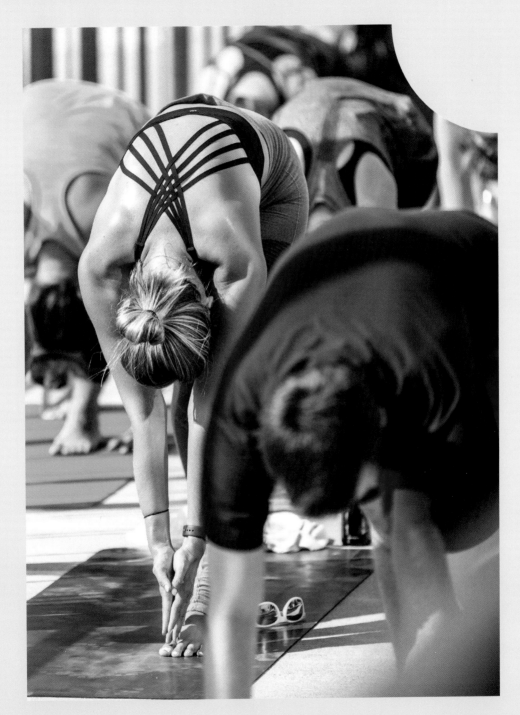

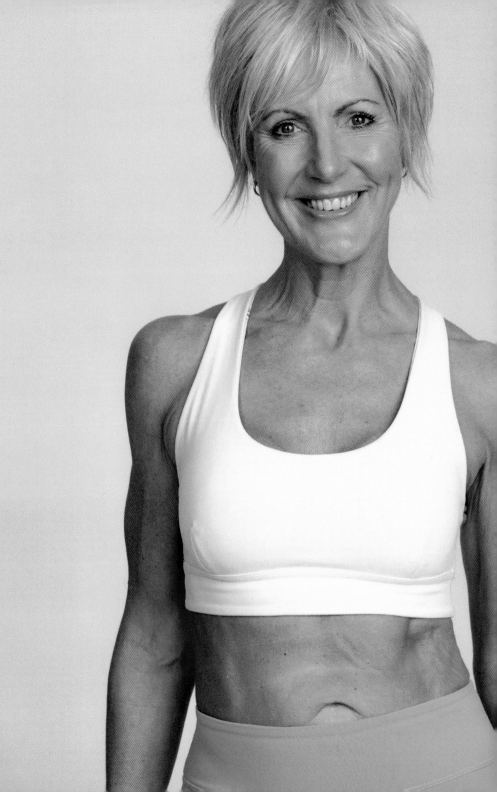

CHAPTER 8

POSITIVITY

BELIEVING YOU CAN BE THE BEST VERSION OF YOU

Henry Ford said if you believe you can, or believe you can't; you're probably right.

Does any of this sound like you?

I **NEVER** lose any weight when I diet.

I **DON'T** like exercise.

I **CAN'T** give up wine/cake/sugar.

I have had a binge weekend so it's all ruined, I **SHOULD** start again on Monday.

I **HAVE TO** start eating healthier food.

If so, it is important to see that these are all limiting beliefs that will hinder you in pursuit of your goals. This negative language also creates a self-fulfilling prophecy. We need to change the language you use to reflect positive and enabling beliefs.

REPLACE

I never with **I WILL**

I can't with **I CAN**

I don't with **I AM LUCKY TO**

I should with **I AM GOING TO**

I have to with **I GET TO.**

Instead of closing down possibility, you are opening it up.

For me, I wanted to celebrate turning 60, to see it as the start of something, not the beginning of the end. I could have focused on my wrinkles or my creaky knees and told myself "What does it matter what I look like at 60?". If I had thought it too late to start something new, I would have a completely different perspective. I would never have set out on my challenge for fear of failing.

> *Believe in yourself and your ability to make healthier choices. You're stronger than you think. You have the power to transform your life within touching distance at all times.*

Developing a positive mindset is a valuable skill that can significantly improve your overall well-being and outlook on life. This is going to play a large part in achieving your fitness goals. Have any of you ever done a strengths finder exercise? I have used Clifton Strengths in the past to understand the dynamic I brought to my work team. It's a great thing to do as it puts a spotlight on your greatest strengths and when is that ever a bad thing? One of my top 5 traits was positivity. Here are some ways to make sure you go into this challenge absolutely brimming with the stuff.

DITCH THE INNER CRITIC

If you catch yourself listening to your internal critic, stop! Would you constantly tell your friend negative things about them? Of course not! So why do it to yourself? Treat yourself with the same kindness and understanding that you offer to others. A Chinese proverb says, "Your thoughts become your words, the words influence your actions, the actions become a habit and your habits become your character, your character determines the outcome of your destiny". So instead of listening to the critic…

GIVE YOURSELF A PEP TALK IN THE MIRROR

I was taught that if you repeat something three times over out loud, your brain creates new neural pathways in order to remember the words. This is a technique called neurolinguistic programming. Repeating positive affirmations or statements re-programmes negative thought patterns and replaces them with empowering ones. Positive affirmations trump negative self-talk. Repeat phrases that reinforce your self-worth and self-appreciation. Remember your achievements and challenges that you have overcome. Then consider all of the accomplishments, skills, capabilities and qualities that helped you succeed in the past.

With this in mind, create a positive mantra in the present tense that represents how you will feel at the end of your goal. Here is an example, but feel free to adapt if you want something more appropriate for you.

Repeat after me.

I am happy and confident and I achieve everything I set out to do

I am happy and confident and I achieve everything I set out to do

I am happy and confident and I achieve everything I set out to do

MANIFEST SUCCESS

If you want to try taking this one step further, there is the 369 method. Supposedly created by Nikola Tesla, this combines numerology with the Law of Attraction. This involves writing down your positive affirmation 3 times when you wake up, 6 times at midday and 9 times before you go to bed, for 3 days. The repetition is going to reinforce your intention and is believed to signal to the universe your desire to bring thoughts into reality. There are lots of instances where people say it's worked for them – so why not give it a go?

SURROUND YOURSELF WITH RADIATORS NOT DRAINS

Do you know the people who you can't wait to see because you always feel energised after seeing them? Or the ones who uplift and support you whatever you're up to? These are your radiators. Spend as much time as you can with them!

The drains? These are the negative people who drain your energy and outlook. You don't need them right now; you're on a mission!

Share your goals with the radiators as they are going to love seeing you succeed.

Be picky who you follow on social media. Reduce your consumption of negative news or media, cruel gossip or lifestyles that are unaffordable, unachievable and frankly unbelievable. You only get to see very polished, filtered versions of these lives. It can increase feelings of anxiety and make you feel inadequate as you juggle the stresses of day-to-day life.

I try to post photos of me with messy hair doing a workout at home after having crawled out of bed and into my gym kit. After all, that is real life. Of course, I also enjoy posting photos of myself looking scrubbed-up for a night out.

I recently caught myself looking critically at my skin on a video compared to another person's on Instagram. I swiftly reminded myself that "comparison is the thief of joy!" I can only be the best version of myself, so that should be the benchmark.

CELEBRATE YOUR SUPER POWERS

I have already mentioned that many years ago I did a strengths finder test as part of my self-improvement journey. They are quite cheap to do online and the idea is to find those skills that you are brilliant at. When I found out about them, I decided to grow and develop those and make them superpowers rather than focus on things I was average at.

I had spent too long comparing myself to my bosses and limiting belief in myself just because I didn't excel in the same ways they did. If you are interested, mine were POSITIVITY, STRATEGY, WOO (Winning Others Over) INDIVIDUALISATION (treating each person as unique) and MAXIMISER (making things the best they can be).

Anyway, this proved to be a life changing moment as I realised that I was totally unique, just as you are too. The only thing I can do is try to be the best version of me.

If you don't want to do a test, why not ask your friends and family to list your 3 best qualities. I am sure there will be some that crop up over and over again. These are the things people love about you and they will be your superpowers. Never compare yourself, start celebrating being you and flex those superpowers like never before. Find ways of using them to support your goals.

LAUGH IN THE FACE OF ADVERSITY

I always laughingly say to expect the unexpected. Be gentle with yourself when things don't work out like you hoped. If you don't do well at an exercise the first time, or have another week of the dial on the scales not moving, put it down as a blip and a lesson to learn from.

Challenges and failures are opportunities for growth. Embrace the belief that you can learn and improve from your experiences during this process. Thomas Edison, the inventor of the lightbulb, famously said "I have not failed. I've just found 10,000 ways that won't work". His message is simple: keep going and your light will shine brightly.

BE BODY POSITIVE

People often comment on my shoulders, for which I have genetics to thank. My fabulous Aunt Angela (my dad's sister) is 79 and she looks incredible with shapely shoulders and arms. My lovely daughter has inherited the same genes. I spent a long time as a young woman (and in my 40's) longing for slim legs when my genetics always meant mine were sturdier. But I have always had shapely arms.

Work out the bits of your body you love and give them some appreciation. We can find the best exercises to improve the bits you don't like so much. I think accepting the gift of a body you have been given but keeping it in the best shape you can is the path to inner peace. If I could talk to my 20 year old self or even my 40 year old self, this is what I would tell them. Celebrate yourself and never, ever compare!

FIND THE EXERCISE YOU LOVE.

Make time for activities that bring you joy and fulfilment. I mentioned before that I never really enjoyed sport until I discovered I liked table tennis and badminton. I also know that any regime that involves jumping around to my favourite music, whether its Zumba, Dancercise or even HIIT, makes exercise more enjoyable for me. Physical activity can boost your mood and positivity. It is not a punishment, it's a celebration of what your body can do. Remember to use positive language. There's a fitness routine for everyone and I hope you will enjoy some of the exercises I share. Remember, there are so many ways online to try things without making a huge commitment.

CREATE YOUR POSITIVITY PLAYLIST

I have one. Songs that make my heart swell and uplift me. I used to listen to this on the tube or the drive to work to make me feel on top of the world and ready to slay the day.

Some of mine include...

- Mr Blue Sky – ELO
  (Makes me feel its sunny when it's not.)
- This is ME – The Greatest Showman
  (A reminder to be myself and not compare myself to others.)
- Lovely Day – Bill Withers
  (Because of course, it was going to be a lovely day!)
- Tonight's Going to be a Good Night – Black Eyed Peas
  (Because of course... It's going to be a good night!)

I also find music is a big part of enjoying exercise. When I run, I have a 180 bpm (beats per minute) playlist that matches the pace I run at which makes things feel so much easier. For HIIT, bouncy dance tracks keep me feeling high energy.

BE GRATEFUL EVERY DAY

Keep a gratitude journal by your bed. Before you sleep, write down the things that you are grateful for. These can be major or minor. A promotion at work, for example, or just that you had a lovely chat on the phone with your mum. Both are worthy of feeling gratitude. You will sleep better, wake up with a positive mindset and have a record to look back on of fabulous things better than any diary.

BE YOUR OWN BIGGEST SUPPORTER

Acknowledge and celebrate your achievements no matter how minor they may seem (don't rush out and buy cakes!). Be your own cheerleader. Positive reinforcement will build momentum. Give yourself more carrot (now that is healthy) and less stick.

Developing a positive mindset is an ongoing process, like developing a muscle. But the more you develop it, the easier it becomes until it's second nature. Be consistent and practice. This is not just going to help you with reaching your fitness goal, you will be a happier and more confident person in every way, every day.

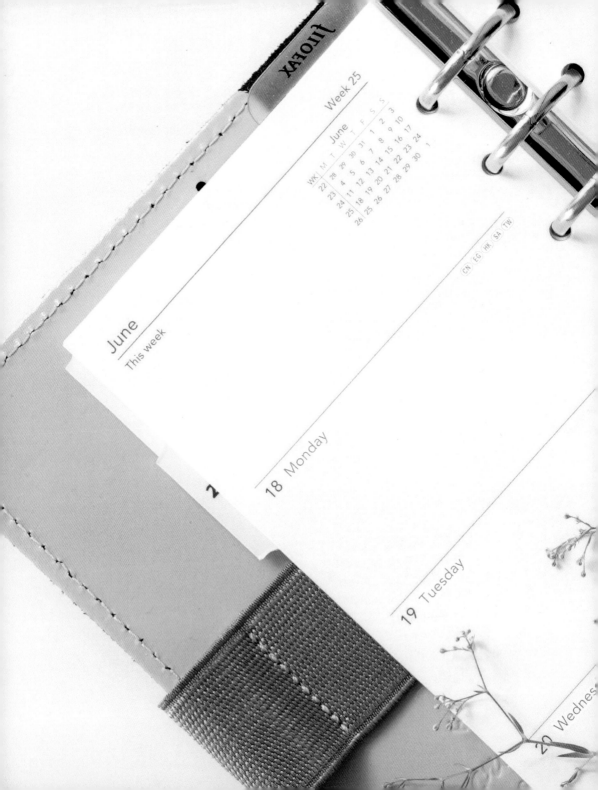

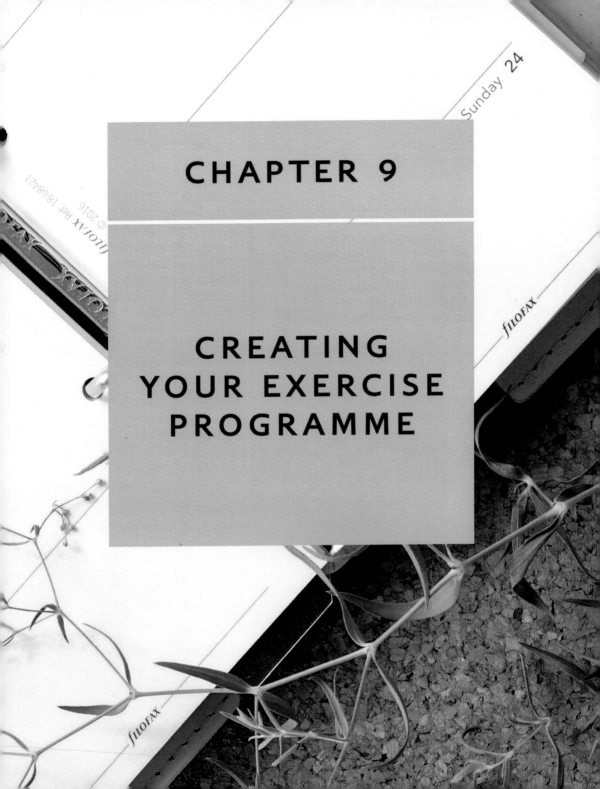

CHAPTER 9

CREATING YOUR EXERCISE PROGRAMME

Everyone asks if I exercise all the time.

I don't!

I do 3–4 hours per week plus walking whenever I can.

For my 60th birthday, my goal was to be at my fittest while reducing body fat and increasing muscle mass. Remember that reducing body fat is crucial for maintaining a healthy weight, reducing the dreaded middle-aged spread and increasing your metabolism. Remember, muscle burns more energy than fat.

Here's a typical weekly timetable:

2 hours with my PT, Joss, who pushed me and ensured I was trying new things while teaching me about the exercises I was doing and which muscle groups they worked.

My home workout was 15– 20 minutes of HIIT or Tabata 4 times per week.

I walked 10–15,000 steps per day.

Why did I enjoy this combination?

Higher-intensity exercises, such as running or high-intensity interval training (HIIT) can deliver an immediate calorie burn and a higher metabolic rate afterwards. This is ANAEROBIC exercise.

Low intensity exercises like walking can be sustained for longer durations, still resulting in an overall fat burn. This is AEROBIC exercise.

Before I share routines that I did at home, here are the benefits of walking, HIIT and Tabata that I learned.

WALKING

Did you know the concept of walking '10,000 steps a day' originated in Japan? The challenge was first created to sell step counters in the lead up to the Tokyo Olympics in 1964, although there was no real evidence to support this target at the time.

Low intensity exercise like walking primarily taps into the body's fat stores for energy, utilising fat as a fuel source. Making walking part of your daily routine contributes to a reduction in body fat percentage over time.

150 minutes of moderate-intensity walking or 75 minutes of vigorous-intensity walking per week is recommended by health guidelines as a minimum. Broken down, this equates to about 30 minutes of walking on most days of the week.

If you want to reduce your body fat percentage more dramatically, you need to increase this. I increased my walking to 10,000 steps per day, minimum, in order to accelerate fat burning. I quickly noticed my legs slimming down.

At my pace, 10,000 steps is a minimum of 1 hour 15 minutes. I walk everywhere I can, as this is a big chunk of time to find in one go, especially if you are working or busy. I would walk to my local shops if I needed something instead of using the car, always choosing the stairs over a lift and being the person who offers to get coffee for others. This all added up.

I won't let rain be an excuse. I got a great rainproof coat or took an umbrella! There's no such thing as bad weather, just the wrong clothes. The smell of the grass or the ground after rain is to be savoured and it is never quite as busy.

If you want to increase the intensity of walking as an exercise, you can try the following:

- Walking uphill or on an incline will increase the benefits of walking as it engages a greater number of muscles. This can burn more calories and increases fat burning potential. If you're walking outdoors, hunt out hilly routes or use the incline feature on a treadmill.

- Interval training alternates periods of higher intensity and lower intensity. Incorporating intervals into your walking routine can boost fat burning. If you can, alternate between brisk walking and periods of faster-paced walking or gentle jogging. It will increase your heart rate and calories burnt.

Aside from the health benefits, I discovered the many joys of walking instead of taking the car or underground. I saw fabulous architecture I would normally miss, did more people watching and smiled at fellow pedestrians.

I discovered that without music playing, I appreciated the sounds of nature, the birdsong and the trees whispering as I walked through parks. It became a form of meditation.

HIIT

So why HIIT (High-Intensity Interval Training)? I have always enjoyed aerobic workouts that get my heart pounding. What I particularly like about HIIT is that it's quick! Short bursts of intense exercise are followed by periods of rest or low-intensity activity. For example, you will do 45 seconds of exercise, 15 seconds of rest, then repeat with different exercises for the duration. There are several reasons why HIIT training works and why I believe it worked for me.

This one is worth repeating:
It's quick!

HIIT workouts are very time-efficient and perfect if you're always rushing around like me. They can last between 10 to 30 minutes. I usually do 15–20 minute sessions. Despite them being short and sweet, HIIT sessions really deliver on the following.

CALORIE BURNING AND FAT LOSS

HIIT is great for reducing body fat. The intense bursts of activity followed by short recovery periods increase the body's demand for oxygen. This increases your metabolic rate. Even better, this increased metabolic rate can carry on after the workout, meaning you continue to burn more calories in the hours afterwards.

IMPROVES YOUR CARDIOVASCULAR HEALTH

You will feel your heart rate increase during HIIT, so it will be improving your cardiovascular health. If you haven't done it before, you will get out of breath, but you will find your cardiovascular endurance improves. I have seen my resting heart drop to under 60 with consistent HIIT training.

MUSCLE TONE

HIIT will improve your muscle tone. It won't have the same effect as lifting heavy weights, but the quick and intense nature of HIIT, often using body weight, will lead to lower body fat, revealing more of your newly toned muscles.

VARIETY

If you are going to make exercise a permanent fixture in your life, it needs to keep you interested. HIIT is very versatile and can have many permutations. From bodyweight exercises to sprints, cycling to rowing, at home or in the gym, you can engage different muscle groups. I have been doing it for 5 years and I'm still not bored.

YOU CAN GET EXCITED ABOUT PROGRESS

Your body will adapt quickly to HIIT. It's exciting to realise you're finding it easier and that there's potential for continual progress. You can increase the intensity, duration and try new exercises to keep challenging yourself.

TABATA

Tabata training is a variation of HIIT developed by Japanese scientist Dr. Izumi Tabata and his team. It has the same benefits as HIIT training. The typical structure of a Tabata workout consists of 20 seconds of all-out effort followed by 10 seconds of rest, repeated for a total of 8 cycles, or 4 minutes.

It will normally entail 4 moves repeated 8 times with a minute of rest in between, so it is a 20-minute workout.

Tabata only uses bodyweight and as it has a more rigid structure, it is potentially easier to follow with only 4 exercises per routine.

It builds great cardiovascular health in a very short time.

Tabata is perfect if you are travelling as it can easily be done in a hotel room. For both HIIT and Tabata, you can easily download apps to time yourself at home.

I have kept fairly fit up until now and I am conscious that not everyone will be at the same level. As a result, I am sharing two sets of exercises. One for if you're just starting out and a second more challenging version.

As you progress, you can add weights in the form of dumbbells to most of the exercises in order to enhance the challenge. It's never too late to begin a fitness journey and even small changes in your activity level can have a positive impact on your health and well-being.

However, do consult with a healthcare professional before starting a new exercise programme, especially if you have any underlying health concerns.

"What equipment do I need?"
I hear you ask

Not much! I suggest you have a yoga or non-slip exercise mat, so that exercises lying on the floor are comfortable. I also feel the slight cushioning helps my knee joints.

Some exercises will use a sturdy low table, chair or bench. I have a pair of light dumbbells, but a couple of water bottles will work if you don't have any.

RECOMMENDATIONS ON WHAT TO WEAR

A GOOD SPORTS BRA

Start with a well-fitted sports bra that offers excellent support and minimises movement during exercise. This is especially crucial for activities involving high impact, such as running or HIIT. Aside from your sports bra, comfortable and moisture-wicking underwear is equally important. You can find seamless or moisture-wicking underwear that stays in place and prevents chafing (none of us want that!).

WICKING FABRICS

There are now moisture-wicking fabrics like polyester or nylon blends that draw sweat away from your body, keeping you dry and comfortable. Avoid cotton as it tends to retain moisture.

COMPRESSION LEGGINGS

When it comes to bottoms, leggings or joggers made from stretchy, breathable and wicking materials are a great choice. If you also look for compression fabrics, they can aid circulation too, which helps recovery. Look for high-waisted options that offer support around the middle but ensure a comfortable fit that doesn't dig in. I do like a pocket for a phone or keys, but you get a smoother silhouette without.

A LAYER WHILE YOU WARM UP/STRETCH

Look at breathable and lightweight fabrics like technical tees, tank tops or zip-throughs. Layer for versatility. Start with a moisture-wicking base layer, add a lightweight top and have a breathable jacket or hoodie for cooler weather. This way, you can easily adjust your clothing according to your body's temperature during workouts. I also look out for garments that bridge casual and sportswear, as they will get worn so much more.

A SUPPORTIVE TRAINER

The importance of a good trainer can't be overstated. I have invested in a quality pair (several actually) that are very light, have good support and a lot of bounce to protect my knees as I do HIIT. Whether it's HIIT, running, cross-training or weightlifting, the right footwear provides stability, support and helps prevent injuries. Ensure the shoes fit properly and allow enough room for your toes while providing ample support for your arches and ankles.

NON SLIP, ABSORBANT SOCKS

Find yourself a good cushioned, absorbent cotton trainer liner that doesn't slip into your trainers as you work out – there is nothing more annoying!

RECYCLED FABRICS

A lot of gym wear is made from polyester and nylon, both of which are now readily available as recycled material. Manufacturers are continuously investing in research and development to improve the quality and versatility of recycled fabrics. Advancements in technology have led to the creation of high-performance recycled textiles that have excellent breathability and wicking properties.

As a fun fact, we only have nylon as a result of the USA and Britain working together in the '60s to create fabrics for space travel. Teams in New York and London came up with NY-LON. One useful thing to know for a quiz night.

Are you ready to start your own exercise programme based on what I did at home?

1. Here's the easy ask, walk 10,000 plus steps a day.

2. Commit 15–20 mins 4–5 times per week to exercise in order to see a difference. Book the time in your diary now.

I will be showing you exercises that target different problem areas and show a version to get you started along with a more challenging version for when you progress.

YOUR EXERCISE PROGRAMME

All you have to do is:

Choose if you want to focus on one area or perform a mix of workouts. I will suggest some combinations.

Choose the level you want to do.

Decide between your own pace based on a number of repetitions of the same exercise (reps), HIIT or Tabata.

Routines will take 15–20 minutes depending on your pace, plus allow 5 mins to stretch afterwards.

WHICH BODY PART DO YOU WANT TO FOCUS ON?

ABS-PIRATION TUMMY	THE BUM DEAL THIGHS AND BUM	ARM-AGEDDON ARMS AND SHOULDERS	AERO-DYNAMIC AEROBICS
Crunches	Squat / Prisoner Squat	Press ups	Jumping Jacks
Mountain Climbers	Forward / Reverse Lunge	Tricep Dips	High Knees
Russian Twist	Curtsey Squat	Lat Raises	Burpees
Heel Touches	Glute Bridge / Single Leg Glute Bridge	Shoulder Press	Ice Skaters
Kick Outs	Wall Sit	Shoulder Taps	Jumping Lunges
Bicycles	Step Ups with Knee Lift	Bicep Curl	Frog Jumps
Plank			

TIPS BEFORE YOU START ANY EXERCISE

Think about the muscles you are working

Make sure you intentionally engage and think about the muscles you are working. This is called kinesthesia or body awareness. It increases the mind muscle connection and ensures you get the most out of the exercise. You will also be able to use this on a day-to-day basis, whether sitting or standing in a queue to flex and use muscles.

BREATHING

It's common to find yourself holding your breath when exercising but use it to help perform the move. When you are in the exertion phase of an exercise, breath out through the mouth and inhale as you return to the starting position.

WARM UP

I know I am trying to help you squeeze workouts into your busy day, but ideally try to warm up your body first for a few minutes. If you can, do a few joint rotations.

Begin by gently rotating your joints to increase their mobility. Move your neck in circles (both clockwise and anti-clockwise), rotate your shoulders backward and forward and perform wrist and ankle rotations. This helps lubricate the joints and prepares them for movement.

Try and slowly get your heart rate up and increase blood flow to your muscles, by brisk walking or jogging in place.

Do a couple of dynamic stretches which are slow, controlled stretches that help improve flexibility and loosen muscles. Some examples would be walking lunges and torso twists. Perform each movement for 10–15 repetitions on each side.

STRETCH AFTERWARDS

There are several reasons why stretching after exercise is essential. Post-exercise stretching helps flexibility by elongating muscles and tendons and increasing your range of motion. If you are more flexible, you will improve your workout and reduce the risk of injury both during exercise and in daily life.

Stretching will also alleviate muscle tension and soreness, relaxing the muscles that have been contracting and tightening during exercise, thereby promoting better blood circulation. It will aid in the removal of lactic acid, reducing stiffness and soreness as well as aiding in muscle repair and recovery.

Ever had really aching muscles for two days after a new exercise? That is delayed onset muscle soreness (or DOMS) which is caused by micro tears in the muscles.

Stretching increases blood flow to the muscles, enhancing circulation. This improved blood circulation helps in the efficient distribution of nutrients and oxygen, contributing to better muscle recovery and overall health.

Stretching is essential for good posture. It counteracts the tightening and shortening of muscles that occur during exercise, preventing imbalances that could lead to postural issues and potential injuries.

Stretching post-workout can have a calming effect on the body and mind. If you have been energetic and done 20 mins of HIIT, stretching is a 5 minute pause before you get on with your day. It helps activate the parasympathetic nervous system, promoting relaxation and reducing stress levels.

Hold each stretch for about 15–30 seconds and focus on breathing deeply and relaxing into the stretch.

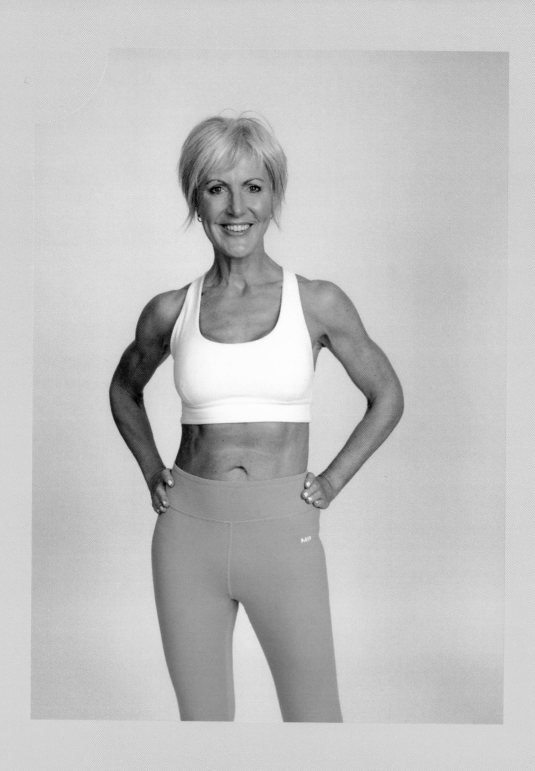

The Exercises

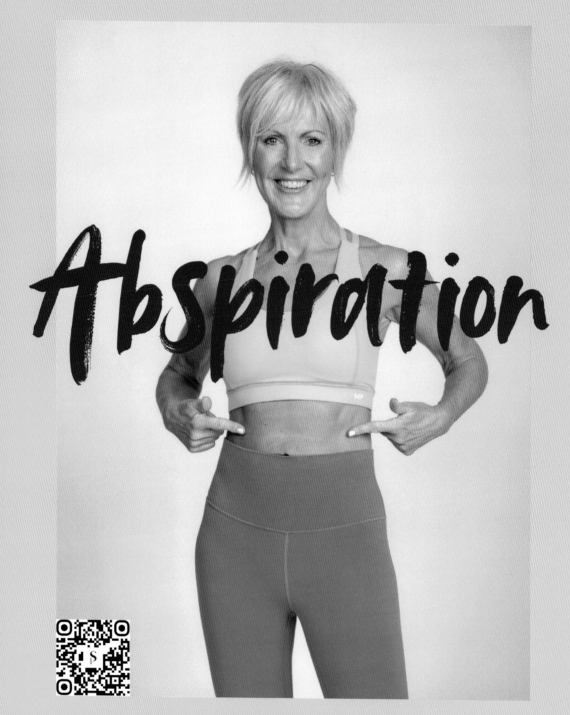

Abspiration

CRUNCHES
Focus on your upper abs

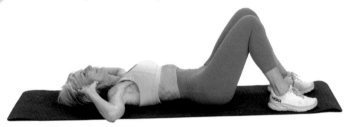

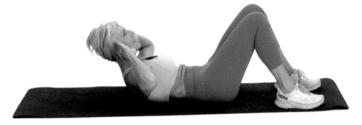

Lie flat on your back, knees bent, feet flat on the floor,
hands just behind your head.

Engage your core and gently lift your head, shoulder blades,
and upper back off the floor, exhaling as you go.

Hold at the top and count to three to maximize muscle engagement.

4

Slowly lower back to floor inhaling ready to repeat.

ASSISTED MOUNTAIN CLIMBERS

Great for cardio and lower tummy

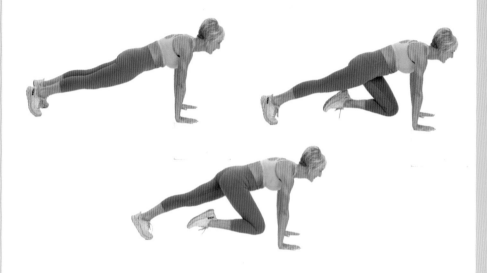

1

Start in plank position with hands on a bench or chair.

2

Bring one knee to chest, then switch legs as quick as you can, avoiding twisting your body.

MADE HARDER

Do the same action with your
hands placed on the ground instead of an elevated platform.

RUSSIAN TWIST

This tightens up your sides

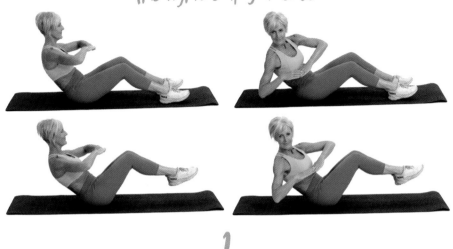

Sit on the floor with your knees bent and your feet flat.

2

Lean back making a 45-degree angle to the floor and loosely clasp hands together.

3

With knees together, feet on the floor, rotate your torso to the right and try to touch the ground, exhale as you do.

4

Pause briefly, then rotate to the left to repeat.

MADE HARDER

From previous start position, raise your feet slightly off the floor and perform as above.

HEEL TOUCHES

This will tighten up your obliques (side muscles) and core

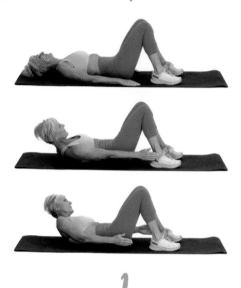

Lie on your back, with knees bent, feet flat on the floor.

Raising your body slightly and tightening your core, reach down your left side to try to touch your left heel. Do not strain your neck, keep in a neutral position.

3

Repeat on the other side, touching your right heel with your right hand, keeping body raised and core tight.

Touch alternate heels for the required count.

KICK OUTS

Great for your lower stomach

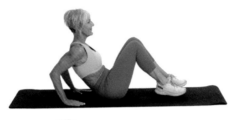

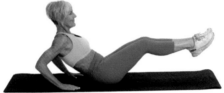

1

Sit on the floor with your knees bent and your feet flat.

2

Lean back making a 45-degree angle to the floor, hands behind you, fingers facing forward.

3

Bring knees to chest.

4

Stretch both legs out in front of you keeping your feet off the ground.

5

Return knees to chest and repeat.

BICYCLES

Works your upper, lower and side abs

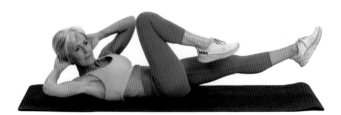

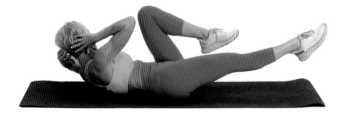

1

Lie down on your back, knees bent, feet on the floor, hip-width apart.

2

Lift your knees to 90 degrees and raise your upper body.

3

Rotate your torso, moving your right elbow and left knee toward each other, other leg extended, exhaling as you do.

4

Inhale and return to starting position, then repeat with other leg.

PLANK

For a flat tummy and strong core

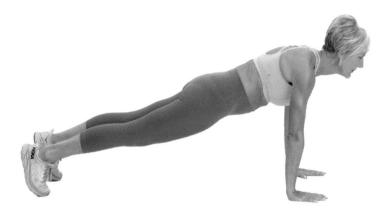

1

Lift your body, supporting it on your hands and balls of feet.

2

Hands should be below your shoulders, body in a straight line.

3

Keep your core muscles engaged.

4

Hold for allotted time.

To make the plank more challenging, support yourself on your elbows.

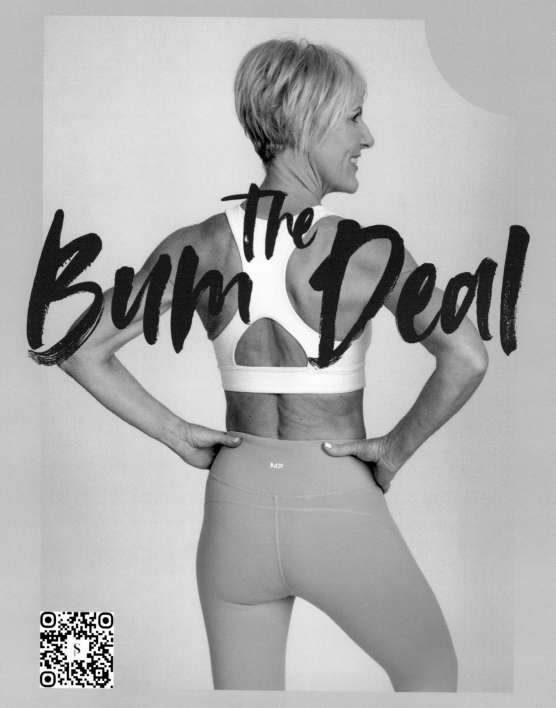

The Bum Deal

SQUAT

Works your bum, thighs and calves

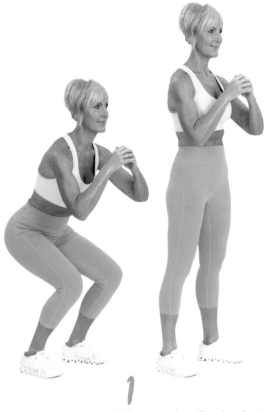

1

Stand with feet shoulder width apart, feet flat, back straight.

2

Lower to a sitting position and hold for 3 seconds.

3

Push through your heels to return to start.

PRISONER SQUAT

For thighs, bum and calves

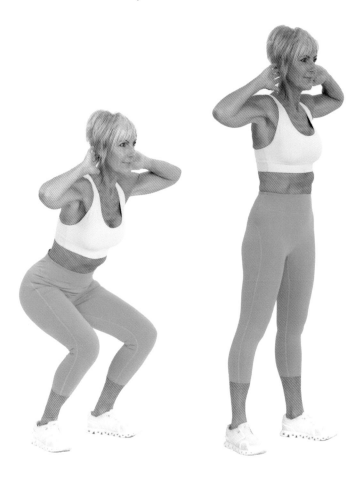

To make the squat more challenging put your hands behind
your head or in the air.

FORWARD LUNGE

Will work your bum, thighs, hamstrings and calves

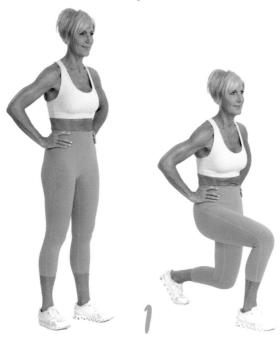

1

Stand with your feet about hip-width apart.

2

Step forward with your right foot until both knees form a 90-degree angle, left knee just above the floor.

3

Push through the heel of your front foot to return to the starting position.

4

Repeat with left leg.

CURTSEY SQUAT

Great for your bum and inner thigh

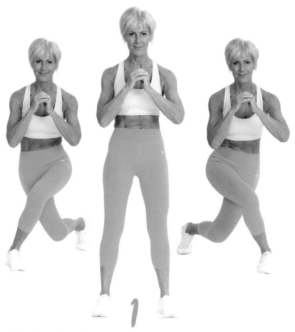

1

Stand with feet shoulder width apart, feet flat, back straight.

2

Step behind with your right foot into a deep curtsey
with front knee at 90 degrees.

3

Push through your heel to return to start and repeat with other leg.

4

You can add weights to increase difficulty.

GLUTE BRIDGE

A focus on lifting your bottom

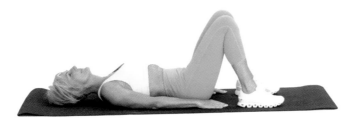

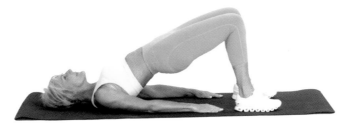

1

Lay down on your back with your knees bent and your feet flat on the ground, hip-width apart and arms by your sides.

2

Squeeze your glutes and your abs and lift hips toward the ceiling as high as possible keeping body in a straight line.

3

Squeeze the glutes as tightly as you can and hold for two seconds.

4

Slowly lower the hips down to the floor and repeat.

SINGLE LEG GLUTE BRIDGE

Increases the work on one side

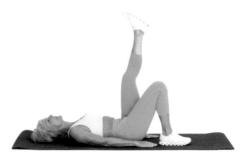

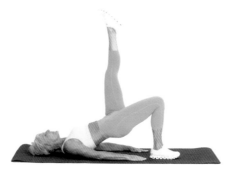

1

Start with hips raised as the glute bridge, then lift left leg and straighten to point it at the ceiling. Hold for 2 seconds.

2

Holding this leg position, lower hips to the floor, then raise to repeat movement exhaling as you go.

3

When reps are complete, change legs and repeat on other side.

WALL SIT

Hold this for thighs, bum, calves and core

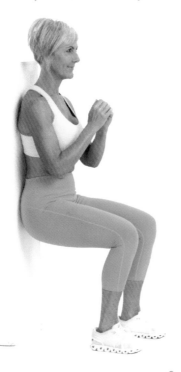

1

Put your back against a wall, feet shoulder width and slide your back down the wall until knees are bent at 90 degrees and directly above your ankles.

2

Keep your back flat against the wall and hold the position.

3

Slide slowly back up the wall to a standing position.

STEP UPS WITH KNEE RAISE

This will really work your thighs

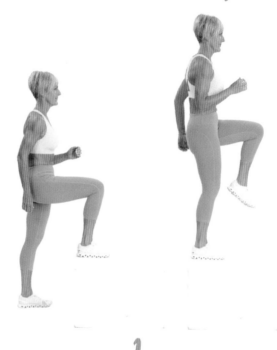

1

Facing a bench or a step, step up onto the bench and as you step, drive the opposite knee up in the air bending at the hip. Exhaling as you push up. Swing opposite arm to keep your balance.

2

When supporting leg is straight not locked, bring the knee back to starting position and then step off the bench back down to standing position.

3

Repeat with opposite leg.

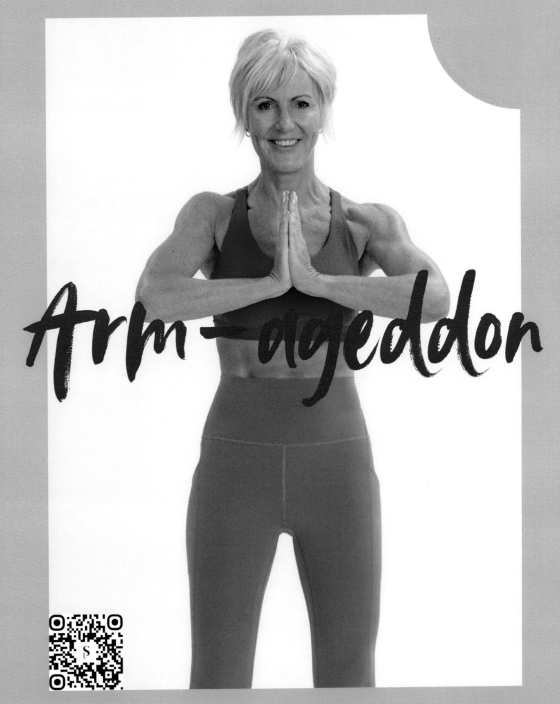

Arm-ageddon

ASSISTED PUSH UP
For chest or pectoral muscles and triceps

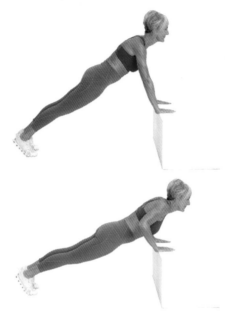

This can be done off a table or bench. The lower it is, the harder it is.

With hands wider than shoulder width apart on bench, stretch legs out straight out behind you, resting on your toes with body in a straight line.

3

Inhale as you lower your body, bending your elbows to 90 degrees, then push back, to straighten arms without locking, bringing your body back to starting position, exhaling as you do.

PUSH UP
To work chest muscles harder

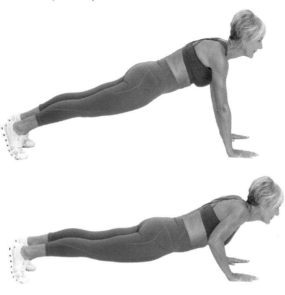

Lie down with your chest and stomach flat on the floor. Legs should be straight out behind you, resting on your toes and your palms flat on the floor at chest level.

Exhale as you push from your hands to straighten arms without locking, bringing your torso, chest, and thighs off the ground.

3

Pause in the plank position, keeping core engaged for a second, then slowly lower back to your starting position, inhaling as you do.

TRICEP DIPS

To banish the bingo wing

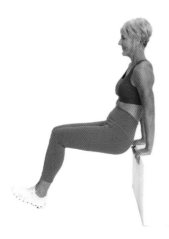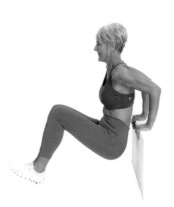

1

Sit on a sturdy bench or chair, with hands facing forward, press into palms slide forward so your bottom just clears the edge.

2

Lower until elbows are bent between 45 and 90 degrees inhaling as you go.

3

Push back up slowly until your arms are almost straight, exhaling as you go, then repeat.

4

To increase difficulty, straighten your legs out in front of you.

LAT RAISE
For a toned back

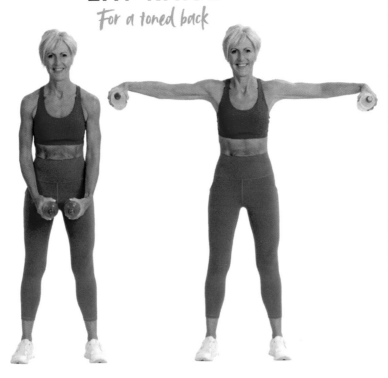

1

Stand with feet hip width apart, knees slightly bent.

2

Hold weights with slight bend in elbows and shoulder blades pushed together.

3

Raise the weights sideways slowly to shoulder height, pause, then lower slowly.

SHOULDER PRESS
For shapely shoulders

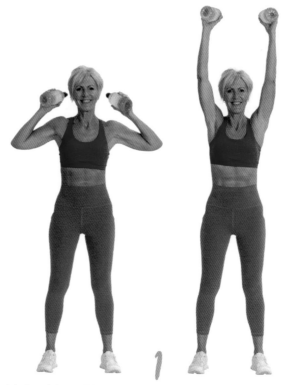

1
Stand with feet hip width apart, chest up and weights held at shoulders.

2
Bracing your core, push the weights directly upwards until arms are almost straight, weights directly above your shoulders.

3
Slowly lower the weights back to shoulders, pause, then repeat.

ASSISTED PLANK WITH SHOULDER TAP

For a flat tummy, strong core and shapely shoulders

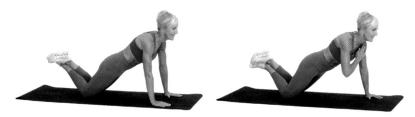

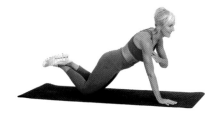

1
Start in assisted plank position, knees on the floor, your body in a straight line.

2
Tap your left shoulder with your right hand.

3
Return your hand to the floor then lift your left hand to tap your right shoulder.

4
Alternate tap each shoulder avoiding rotating your body.

PLANK WITH SHOULDER TAP

For a flat tummy, strong core and shapely shoulders

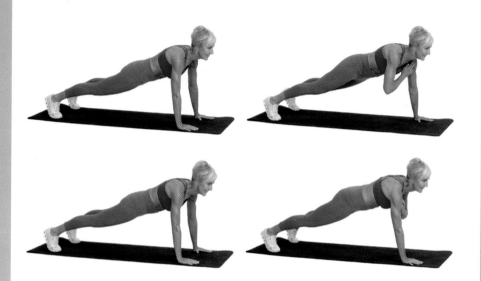

Start in plank position on the floor, your body in a straight line from shoulders to feet.

2

Alternate tap each shoulder avoiding rotating your body.

BICEP CURLS

Tones the biceps at the front of your arm

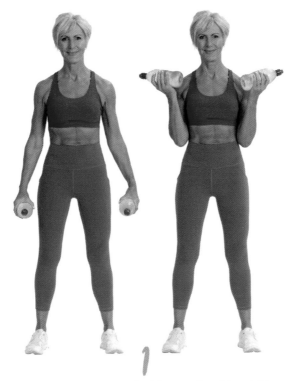

1

Hold a weight in each hand with your feet hip width apart
and arms at your side.

2

Keep your knees slightly bent and with palms facing forward,
curl both arms upward to shoulder level.

3

Slowly lower the weight back down and repeat.

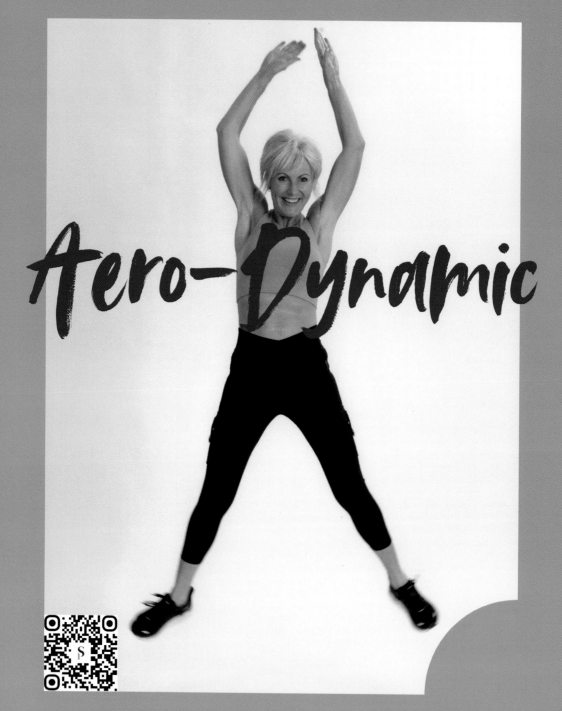

Aero-Dynamic

JUMPING JACKS

This will get your heart pumping as you're jumping

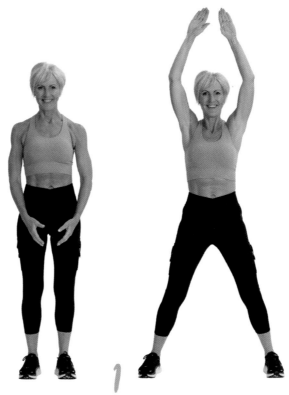

Start with arms at your side, elbows straight, and feet together.

Jumping feet apart and lift your arms over your head exhaling as you do.

3

Bring your hands back down by your side and jump feet back together as you inhale.

HIGH KNEES

This is not only a great cardio vascular exercise but will use your lower stomach muscles

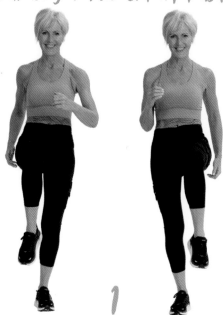

1

Stand with feet together.

2

Start to run on the spot using your core to lift your legs up to hip height for allotted time.

3

Pump your arms as you do.

4

To increase difficulty put your hands behind your head or in the air.

ASSISTED BURPEE
A great full body exercise

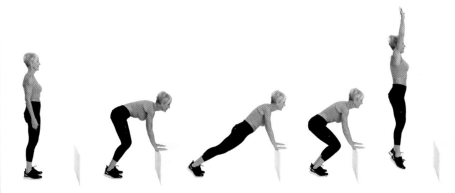

1
Stand facing a bench, chair or table, feet hip width apart.

2
Put both hands on the support, shoulder width apart,
bending knees, then jump legs back so body is straight from shoulder
to ankle, exhaling as you do.

3
Spring legs back in, then straighten up, and jump vertically with hands
up in the air, inhaling as you do this.

4
When you land repeat the move.

BURPEE
Full body workout

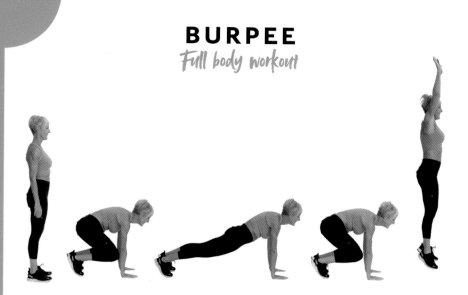

1
Stand with feet hip with apart.

2
Drop into a squat, then supporting your body with hands under shoulders, kick feet back into the plank position. Jump the feet back into a squat, then from there jump in the air with hands above the head.

3
Drop hands to sides and repeat.

(Depending on who is instructing this can be called a half burpee. To add difficulty, you can drop to a press up from the plank position to make this more challenging)

SKATERS

Works inner and outer thighs

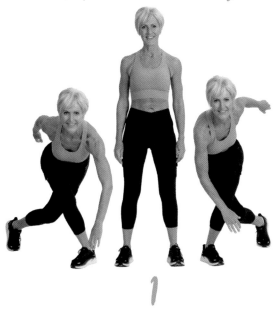

1

Stand feet shoulder-width apart, on the balls of your feet,
with a slight flex in knees.

2

Pushing off one foot, jump sideways onto the other foot, bending the
landing knee and swinging the other foot back diagonally.

3

Swing the opposite arm to the landing foot across your body like a skater.

4

Pause, then reverse the move to hop back onto the other foot,
landing with a bent knee, then keep repeating for the set.

JUMPING LUNGES

A challenging workout for your thighs and bum

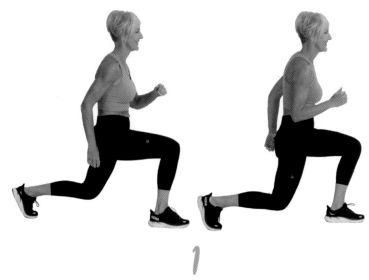

1

Step forward into a deep lunge, lean slightly forward, keeping core tight.

2

Drive both feet into the floor and spring upwards, inhaling,
and quickly switch over to land with the other leg forwards using
your arms to help propel you.

3

As you land, bend the knee to land softly, exhaling as you do, and make sure
your front knee is not beyond your front foot.

4

Drop to a deep lunge position and repeat.

If this feels difficult, try walking lunges and then build up to these.

FROG JUMPS

An explosive exercise for your bum and thighs

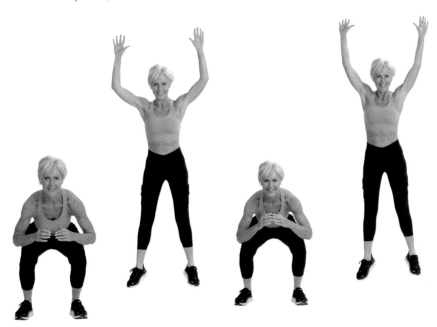

1

Stand with feet just wider than hip width apart and hands by your side.

2

Squat down so knees are bent to 90 degrees, swinging arms back, then spring up into the air using arms to propel you forwards.

3

Land softly, keeping the chest up and bending the knees to go back into the squat position. Repeat.

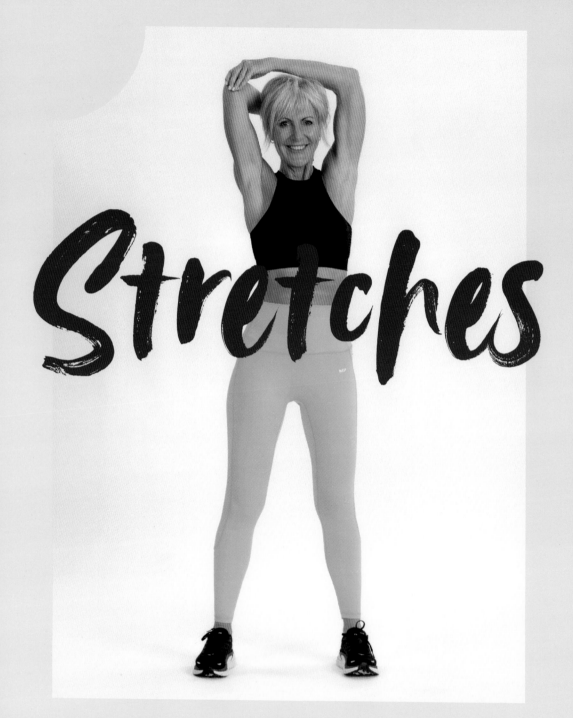

Stretches

FORWARD LUNGE
WITH ROTATION

A dynamic stretch and a great warm up

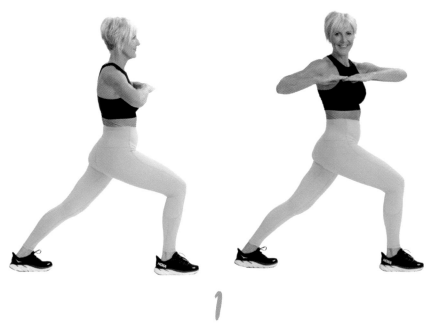

1

Stand with feet hip width apart. With one foot, step forward so that both legs are bent at 90 degrees, back knee close to the floor.

2

Hands are raised in front of chest, and elbows shoulder height. Twist torso in direction of supporting knee as far as comfortable, hold for a moment, then return to centre.

3

Step back to starting position and repeat other leg.
Do this 3 times each side.

QUADRICEP STRETCH

Stretching the front of your thighs

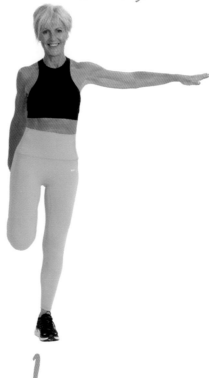

1

Stand upright, weight on right leg, knees together.
Use a chair or the wall for balance if needed.

2

Bring the left foot up towards your bottom and use
the left hand to pull it close to the body.

3

Hold for 15 to 30 seconds, then repeat, switching legs.

TRICEPS STRETCH
Stretching the backs of the arms

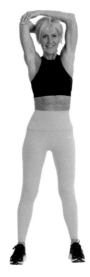

1
Stand straight, feet shoulder-width apart.

2
Bring your left elbow straight up, bending your arm,
so elbow is close to the head.

3
Taking the left elbow with your right hand, pull it toward your head,
with light pressure to feel a stretch in the back of the arm.

4
Hold 15 to 30 seconds, then switch arms.

PECTORAL AND DELTOID STRETCH

Chest and shoulders

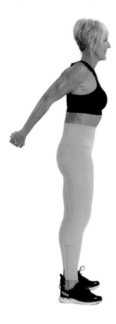

Stand with your feet hip-width apart, brace your core
and push shoulder blades together.

Extend your arms behind your back, clasp your hands together,
push through the hands and slowly lift up.

3

Hold for 15–30 seconds then lower.

HAMSTRING STRETCH

Stretching the backs of your legs

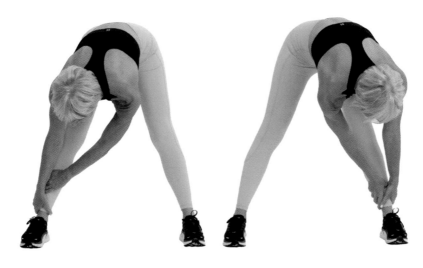

1

Stand with your feet just wider than hip-width apart.

2

Bend forward at the hips and reach towards your toes with both hands.
You feel a slight stretch at the back of your legs.

3

Reach to grab one ankle with both hands, and breathe,
trying to deepen the stretch.

4

Hold for 15 to 30 seconds, then repeat on other leg.
Slowly uncurl up to stand.

COBRA STRETCH

This will stretch out your abdomen

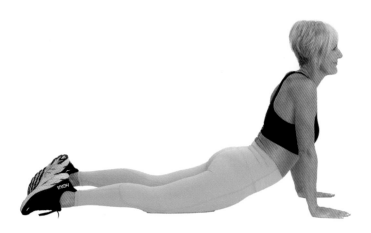

1

Lie face down, legs stretched out and bring hands underneath the shoulder blades.

2

Push off to lift your upper body, straightening arms, looking slightly forward and up.

3

Hold for 15–30 seconds then slowly lower down.

GLUTE STRETCH

Stretches the muscles in your bottom

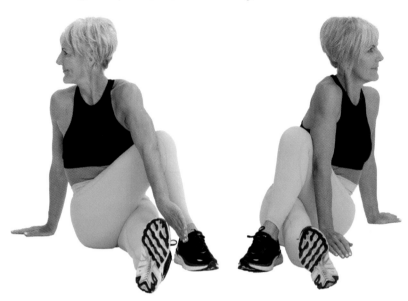

Sit on the floor with your legs straight in front of you, chest up.

Bend your right knee and cross it over your left leg.

3

Twist your torso to the right and reach your left hand
over to touch the floor, keeping back upright. Gently push your right knee
with your left elbow to stretch the gluteus muscle. Hold 15–30 seconds
then repeat on other side.

ABS-PIRATION
A TUMMY BLAST

For 15 minutes
(I did this every day!)

- Mountain climbers x 20
- Crunches x 20
- Kick-outs x 20
- Bicycles x 20
- Heel touches x 20
- Plank 30 seconds
- Repeat 3 times

ARM-AGEDDON
UPPER BODY BLAST

For 15 minutes with a 3kg weight,
or 1L bottle of water (1kg)

- Assisted press ups x 15
- Lat raises x 20
- Shoulder taps x 10 each side
- Shoulder press x 20
- Tricep dips x 15
- Repeat 3 times

THE BUM DEAL
BUM AND THIGH BLAST

For 15 minutes

- Squat x 20
- Forward lunge x 10 each leg
- Glute bridge x 20
- Curtsey squat x 10 each side
- Step ups x 20 in total
- Wall sit x 30 seconds
- Repeat 3 times

HIIT

If you are a new starter, I suggest you do the below for 30 seconds of exercise and 10 second rest which will take around 14 minutes.

You can then progress to 45 seconds of exercise and 15 seconds rest for a 20 minute workout.

HIIT WORKOUT 1 FOR 20 MINS

 Mountain climbers
45 seconds
Rest 15 seconds

 Forward lunges
45 seconds
Rest 15 seconds

 Squats
45 seconds
Rest 15 seconds

 Shoulder taps
45 seconds
Rest 15 seconds

 Jumping jacks
45 seconds
Rest 15 seconds

 Glute bridge
45 seconds
Rest 15 seconds

 Assisted press ups
45 seconds
Rest 15 seconds

 Bicycles
45 seconds
Rest 15 seconds

 High knees
45 seconds
Rest 15 seconds

 Tricep dips
45 seconds
Rest 15 seconds

Repeat once

HIIT

HIIT WORKOUT 2

 Skaters
45 seconds
Rest 15 seconds

 Heel touches
45 seconds
Rest 15 seconds

 Burpees
45 seconds
Rest 15 seconds

 Lat raises
45 seconds
Rest 15 seconds

 Frog jumps
45 seconds
Rest 15 seconds

 Shoulder taps
45 seconds
Rest 15 seconds

 Russian twist
45 seconds
Rest 15 seconds

 Jumping lunges
45 seconds
Rest 15 seconds

 Reverse lunges
45 seconds
Rest 15 seconds

 Wall sit
45 seconds
Rest 15 seconds

Repeat once

TABATA

WORKOUT 1 TAKES 16 MINUTES

 Forward lunges
20 seconds
10 seconds rest
Repeat 8 times
1 minute rest

 Glute bridge
20 seconds
10 seconds rest
Repeat 8 times
1 minute rest

 Shoulder taps
20 seconds
10 seconds rest
Repeat 8 times
1 minute rest

 Crunches
20 seconds
10 seconds rest
Repeat 8 times
1 minute rest

WORKOUT 2 TAKES 16 MINUTES

 Assisted press ups
20 seconds
10 seconds rest
Repeat 8 times
1 minute rest

 Curtsey lunges
20 seconds
10 seconds rest
Repeat 8 times
1 minute rest

 Bicycles
20 seconds
10 seconds rest
Repeat 8 times
1 minute rest

 Wall sit
20 seconds
10 seconds rest
Repeat 8 times

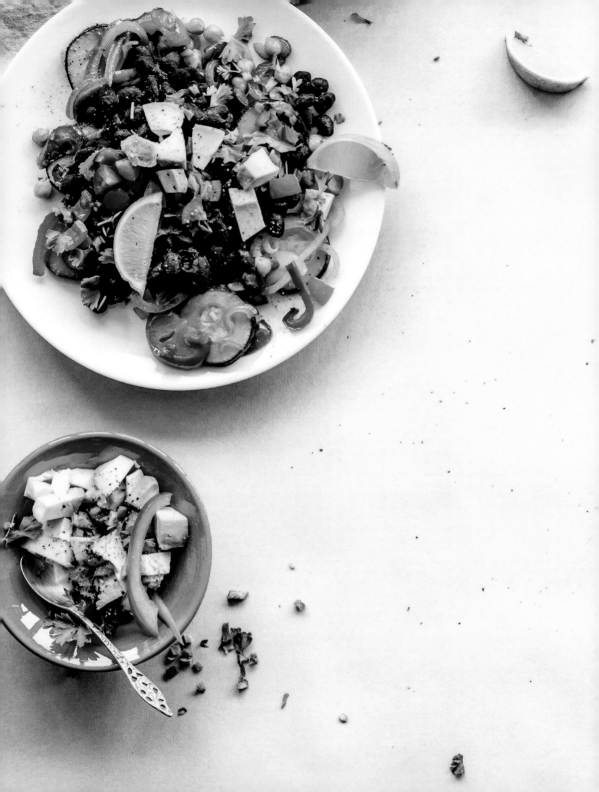

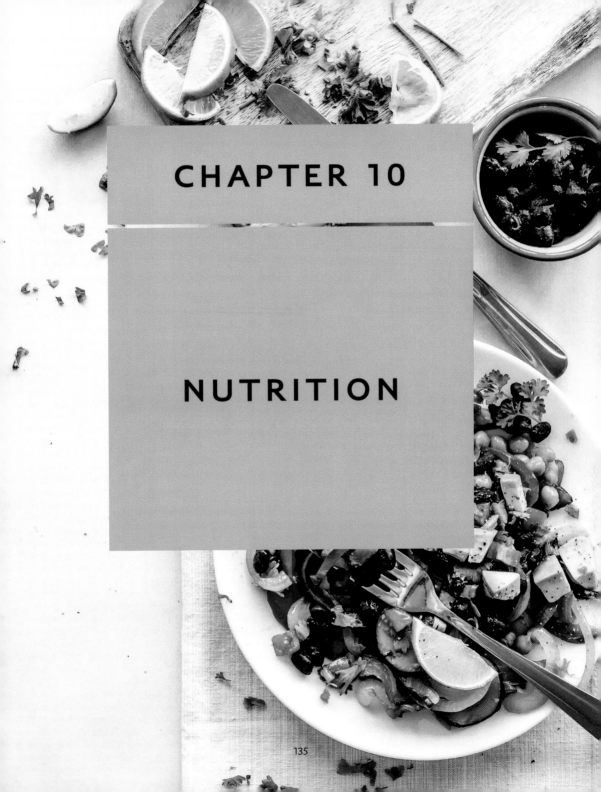

CHAPTER 10

NUTRITION

You can't exercise yourself out of a bad diet.

In order to lose 14lbs and 5% of my total body fat in 90 days, I had a pretty strict plan. Still, I knew it had an end date and so I went into the challenge knowing that I could stick it out for a short period of time.

I needed to have a calorie deficit of 300–400 calories per day in order to reach my goals in the time I had set. There are several apps available that can help you calculate your calorie requirements based on age and height. For me, without doing any exercise, I need around 1700 calories, so my 300–400 calorie deficit meant that without any exercise, I could have 1350 to 1400 calories. Any activity increased that.

I cut out sugar in all forms: sucrose, fructose (in fruit) and lactose (in dairy).

To reduce fat and maintain muscle I needed to eat 0.75g – 100g of protein per kg of body weight.

I drank 2L of water per day and consumed no alcohol. A quick hack, wine is my nemesis, so I drank water from a wine glass in the evening. If you go sparkling you can pretend it's champagne!

I kept a food journal of everything I ate and quickly realised how frequently I had been adding calories through snacking.

I tried (I wasn't 100% perfect) to avoid scrolling on my phone when eating and consciously ate slower, so that I appreciated the food I was consuming and wasn't eating in a fog.

I cooked 90% of the time from fresh ingredients. This ensured that I knew what I was eating and allowed me to appreciate food so much more.

As I am nearly always time short and, as previously revealed, not very patient, most of the recipes I made were ready in 20–25 minutes. I also avoided eating after 7pm.

I emptied my fridge and larder of temptations and planned my meals and snacks in advance to avoid impulsive, unhealthy choices. This made it far easier to stay on track.

For snacky moments I kept ready prepared crudities, flaked salmon, sweet baby cherry tomatoes and cooked squid rings on standby in the fridge. This was so that if I did feel the need, I could easily grab something healthy rather than a biscuit or crisps.

For everyday I stuck to my regime, I mentally gave myself a pat on the back. It helped to remember the feeling of pride as I started anew the following day, knowing how good it felt to succeed.

Faced with external temptation, I pictured myself at my photoshoot, feeling a million dollars with toned abs and a confident smile. All of this helped me say "NO!".

I also learned about the nutritional benefits of the foods I was eating and the positive impact they have on your health. Knowledge can be a powerful motivator.

Importantly, I learned to eat much slower. Why?

DIGESTION

Chewing is the first step in the digestive process. It breaks larger food particles into smaller pieces, helping the gut to process what we eat. Chewing increases saliva production so that you can swallow easily. If large chunks of food enter the digestive tract, they cause digestive problems such as gas, bloating, constipation, adverse reactions, headaches and lowered energy levels. As you chew, digestive enzymes and hydrochloric acid are produced to help break down the food and regulate pH levels. I was prone to heartburn, so this was very helpful to know.

NUTRITION

When food arrives in the stomach in smaller pieces, it is easier for your body to absorb a greater amount of nutrients (including vitamins and minerals).

PORTION CONTROL

I had heard before that it takes about 20 minutes for your brain to let your stomach know that it is full. Therefore, if you are eating slower, it is less likely that you will overeat. My father quotes my grandfather, who always said you should leave the table feeling like you could eat some more (a brilliant tip). If you eat too fast, then overeat, the reverse happens.

PREVENTS BLOATING AND WIND!

Large food chunks that are not properly broken down by eating too fast may start increased fermentation in the gut. This can lead to conditions such as indigestion, bloating, increased gas and constipation, none of which we really want, do we?

I now have a diet that maintains my new weight. If I fluctuate at all, I know how to get back on track.

One thing that isn't really talked about is the fact that carrying less weight around means you will require less calories than you did at the previous weight. You cannot go back to what you were eating before or you will gain weight and undo all of your good work.

To maintain your weight, you need to work out what your new calorie requirement is per day (plus what you burn through exercise).

These are some of the recipes I created by experimenting during the 90 days. They are all quick and simple, as we all have busy lives. They are high in protein, low in carbohydrates and sugars and relatively low calorie.

These recipes serve 2, but they can easily be doubled and if anyone else you're eating with wants to add sourdough bread or replace courgetti with spaghetti, it means it's possible to keep to your stricter diet whilst still being sociable.

MY SHOPPING LIST

PROTEINS

- Eggs
- Smoked mackerel
- Carton of egg whites
- Flaked salmon
- Smoked salmon
- Venison
- Cod
- Tuna steak
- Prawns
- Fresh or cooked chicken breast
- Smoked tofu
- Lean low-fat bacon
- Turkey mince

FLAVOURS

- Fresh herbs
- Lemon
- Vegetable/chicken stock
- Spices
- Sea salt and freshly ground black pepper

VEGETABLES

- Avocado
- Spinach
- Mushrooms
- Canned cherry tomatoes
- Rocket
- Carrots
- Butternut squash
- Beetroot
- Salad
- Shallots
- Canned tomatoes
- Peppers
- Jar of roasted peppers
- Courgettes
- Aubergine
- Red onions
- Cauliflower
- Crushed garlic
- Carbohydrates
- Pre-cooked quinoa
- Pre-cooked lentils
- Celeriac

I should add that there are glaring omissions on my shopping list due to the fact that I have had a very large calcium oxalate kidney stone removed (4cm). Certain vegetables (sweet potato, kale, okra), nuts and spices are very high in oxalate and so unfortunately, I must avoid them. Although many of these foods are super healthy, if I eat them I have to drink a lot more water to compensate.

I have learnt a lot more about nutrition since my 60th birthday as I have been studying personal training. I have also read an incredibly informative book *Let Your Food Be Your Pharmaco-Nutrition* by Dr Paul Clayton which focuses on diet and its impact on ageing caused by inflammation. I have had a high protein, low processed carb diet for years and have oily fish and seafood at least 4 times per week with lots of vegetables. Unbeknownst to me, this has been incredibly good for me combined with exercise. Here are some excerpts from his writings;

"The mid Victorians ate a diet high in nutrient dense foods, copious amounts of fresh vegetables and fruit, pasture raised meats and dairy, eggs, fish, nuts, seeds and legumes. Foods were eaten in season so had as many phytonutrients, vitamins and minerals as possible and the way they grew meant variety throughout the year. Certainly, the working-class people were very active, spending huge amounts of energy doing their day jobs. Men had to walk up to 6 miles to their place of work and women were on their feet most of the day doing domestic chores or jobs in workshops or factories."

"The Blue Zone diet, reduces meat, limits fish and eggs, is high in vegetables and cuts out sugar. The oils used are plant based – with olive oil proving to be consumed heavily by nations with longevity."

In a recent blog he advocates a diet rich in fish as brain food. "Research consistently shows a link between a diet rich in fatty fish and improved cognitive function. There is a haul of publications on the relationship between fish consumption and improved or at least protected cognition, brain volume and structure".

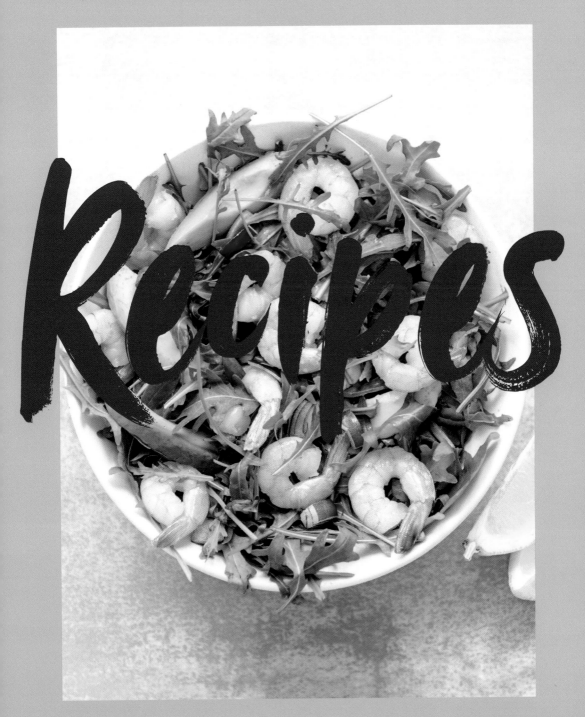

Recipes

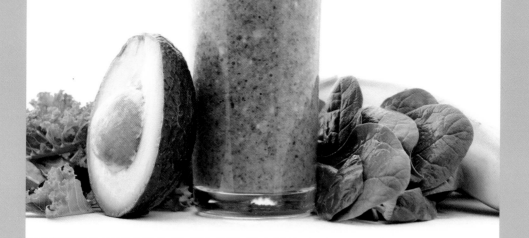

Breakfast

GREEN SMOOTHIE

I was advised by my Personal Trainer, Joss, that this was the perfect way to start the day.

A smoothie is an easy way to get your digestive system working, has lots of fibre and will kick start your metabolism. Celery is considered great for digestion and loaded with antioxidants. It's rich in vitamin A, which boosts immunity, skin health and eye function.

Kale and spinach offer calcium, iron, vitamin A, vitamin C and vitamin K, while kale is packed with flavonoids with anti-inflammatory and anti-carcinogenic properties. The banana and avocado will keep you feeling full through the morning.

The other half avocado will keep in the fridge for a day if you leave the stone in and put it in a container or small bag.

FACT SHEET

Serves 2

Prep time 5 mins

Per portion 198 calories 4g protein 24g carbohydrate

INGREDIENTS

1 banana cut into chunks

2 handfuls of spinach

2 handfuls of kale

1/2 cucumber

1/2 avocado diced

2 celery sticks

Cold water to add to your preference

METHOD

Place all ingredients into a blender and blitz until smooth.

You may want to add salt, pepper or lemon juice to taste.

My alternative "go-to" was a high protein breakfast. Here are a few options, but they can all be combined in different ways.

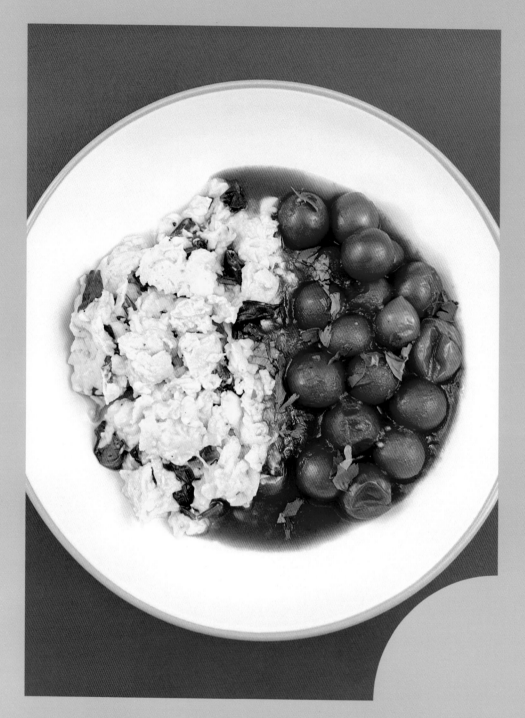

SCRAMBLED EGGS WITH SPINACH AND SAUCY CHERRY TOMATOES

If you scramble the eggs with fresh spinach, you add fibre and vitamins to this breakfast staple. I combine eggs with egg whites to keep the calorific value down and you can't tell the difference. I love a bit of Worcester sauce to add a kick to both mushrooms and tomatoes.

FACT SHEET

Serves 2

Prep time 5 mins

Cooking time 10 mins

Per portion 138 calories 13g protein 7g carbohydrate

INGREDIENTS

200g of tinned sweet cherry tomatoes

Dash of Worcester sauce

Salt and pepper

2 eggs

4 egg whites

A spray of olive oil

Two handfuls of spinach

A sprinkle of chilli flakes if you like spice, or chopped fresh parsley

METHOD

Add tinned tomatoes to a small pan or a microwaveable bowl along with salt, pepper and a dash of Worcester sauce. If cooking on the hob, put on a medium heat to warm through while you prepare the eggs which will be about 5–6 minutes. If you are going to cook in the microwave, this will only take 2 mins on 850W or 1 ½ mins on 1000W, so can be done when the eggs are nearly ready.

Whisk eggs and egg whites in a bowl with salt and pepper.

Spray a medium frying pan with oil and bring to a low-medium heat.

Add the eggs and warm, stirring as they begin to scramble at the bottom of the pan.

When they are almost cooked through, add the spinach, and allow to wilt into the eggs as you stir for about 2 minutes. This is a good time to heat the tomatoes if using the microwave.

When eggs are cooked and spinach is wilted, serve in a shallow bowl with the tomatoes on the side and sprinkle with herbs or chilli flakes if desired.

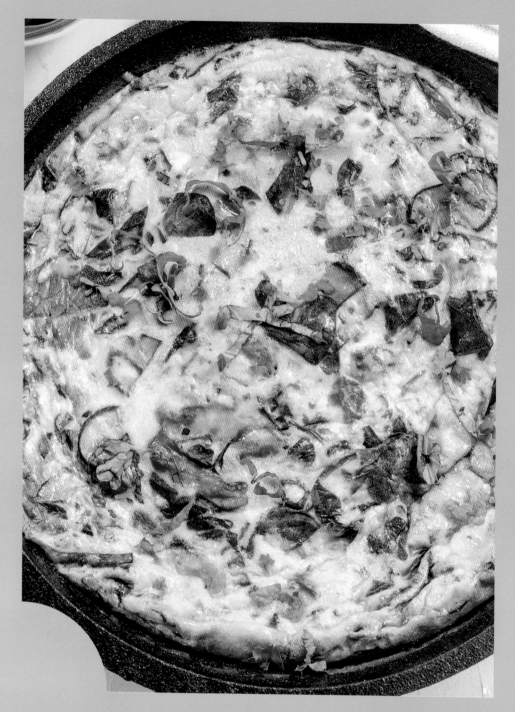

VEGETABLE OMELETTE

I often have an array of vegetables and herbs in the fridge which can get thrown into a vegetable omelette; chopped courgette, peppers fresh or roasted in a jar, asparagus. Variety is the spice of life after all.

FACT SHEET

Serves 2

Prep time 5 mins

Cooking time 12–15 mins

Per portion 182 calories 24g Protein 8g carbohydrate

INGREDIENTS

4 medium eggs

4 egg whites

Fresh dill, parsley and/or mint

Salt and pepper

½ red pepper

1 small shallot

1 baby courgette

Spray olive oil

Handful of baby spinach

Handful of rocket

Handful of chopped mushrooms

METHOD

Whisk eggs and egg whites in a bowl with salt and pepper and chopped herbs.

Finely chop shallot and red pepper, slice courgette and mushrooms.

Heat a medium size frying pan on a low to medium heat and spray base with the olive oil.

Add the red pepper, courgette, mushrooms and shallot to the pan and soften until shallot is transparent. Add the eggs to the vegetables in the pan, then sprinkle over the spinach. Let the eggs cook through and add the rocket to serve.

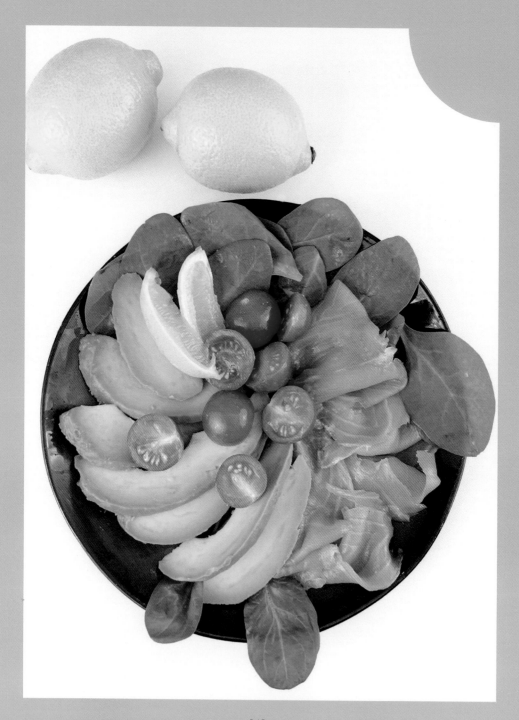

SMOKED SALMON AND AVOCADO

This breakfast is rich in protein, omega 3 and healthy fats. If you want more protein, you can add a poached egg, which works well alongside the other ingredients.

FACT SHEET

Serves 2

Prep time 5 mins

Per portion 248 calories 13g protein 12g carbohydrate

INGREDIENTS

100g of smoked salmon

1 medium avocado

8 cherry tomatoes

2 handfuls of spinach

METHOD

Divide the salmon in two.

Slice the avocado and plate up with salmon and spinach, garnish with halved cherry tomatoes.

Add a few capers or fresh dill if you're feeling fancy!

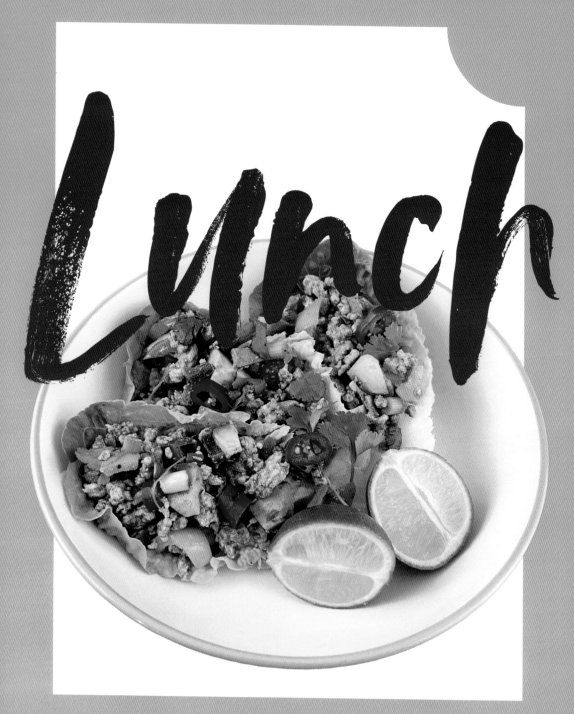

Lunch

LETTUCE CUPS WITH MEXICAN TURKEY MINCE

This is a low carb take on fajitas, using lettuce instead of wraps. It's equally delicious with wraps if you are joined by someone who wants them!

FACT SHEET

Serves 2

Prep time 15 mins

Cooking time 20 mins

Per portion 395 calories 34g protein 12g carbohydrate

INGREDIENTS

Spray olive oil

1 small yellow pepper chopped into 1cm pieces

1 small red pepper chopped into 1cm pieces

½ red onion

250g of 2% fat turkey mince

1 tsp of garlic paste

15g fajita seasoning

3 spring onions sliced

½ ripe avocado cubed

1 fresh chopped red chilli

Small bunch of coriander

Lime juice

1 baby gem lettuce separated into individual leaves

METHOD

In a medium sized frying pan, add spray oil and bring to a medium heat.

Add red onion and chopped red pepper and stir fry to soften for 5 minutes.

Add garlic paste and stir through.

Add turkey mince and cook till no longer pink, breaking up any chunks.

Stir through 15g of fajita seasoning (add more if you like very spicy).

When turkey is cooked add spring onion, avocado, a dash of lime juice, chopped coriander and chilli flakes.

Arrange baby gem leaves on a plate and pile the Mexican turkey mince into the lettuce cups and garnish with more coriander.

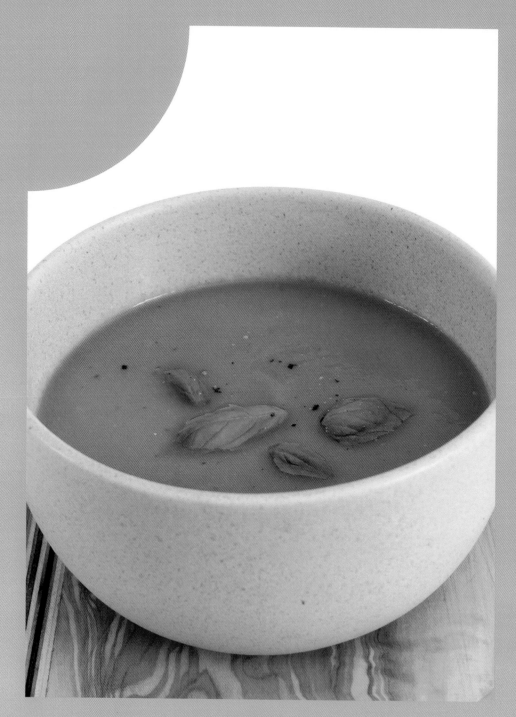

RED PEPPER, CARROT AND TOMATO SOUP

This takes slightly longer to cook than my usual recipes, but you can do a kitchen workout while it's on the hob as its very low maintenance! It keeps well in the fridge so you can be sorted for lunch for a couple of days.

As you add dairy back into your diet it's lovely with milk or cream added.

FACT SHEET

Serves 2

Prep time 5 mins

Cooking time 40 mins

Per portion 130 calories 5g protein 28g Carbohydrate

INGREDIENTS

2 small carrots

½ small white onion

A glug of olive oil

1 red pepper

1 tsp garlic paste

400g tin of tomatoes

300ml vegetable stock

Salt and pepper

Smoked paprika

Fresh basil

METHOD

Finely chop the onion and carrots.

Add olive oil to a medium saucepan and heat before adding chopped onion and carrot. Add lid, stirring regularly to stop sticking.

While these start to soften, de-seed and chop the red pepper into small pieces.

Add to the pan with carrots and onion and continue to soften for about 20 mins.

Add the garlic paste and cook for another minute then add the tin of tomatoes, the stock and paprika.

Stir well and bring to a boil, then simmer for about another 20 mins or until veg is all soft.

Pour into a liquidiser for a really smooth soup or use a hand blender for a chunkier texture.

Add salt and pepper and garnish with fresh basil.

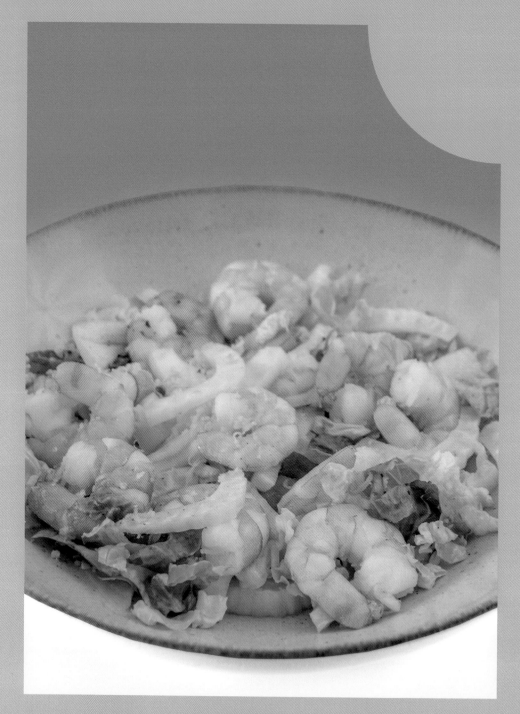

PRAWN, FENNEL AND LEMON SALAD

This is super quick and fresh tasting. Fennel is one of my favourite vegetables whilst you will also notice lots of lemon in my cooking.

I love it! It adds juiciness without any oil.

FACT SHEET

Serves 2

Prep time 5 mins

Per portion 236 calories 50g protein 9g carbohydrate

INGREDIENTS

Small fennel bulb

400g king prawns

1 baby gem lettuce

1 fresh lemon

Salt and black pepper

METHOD

Finely slice the fennel

Chop the lettuce and mix with the fennel and prawns. Add salt and pepper.

Divide between two plates.

Grate lemon zest over the salad then juice the lemon, pouring over the two salads.

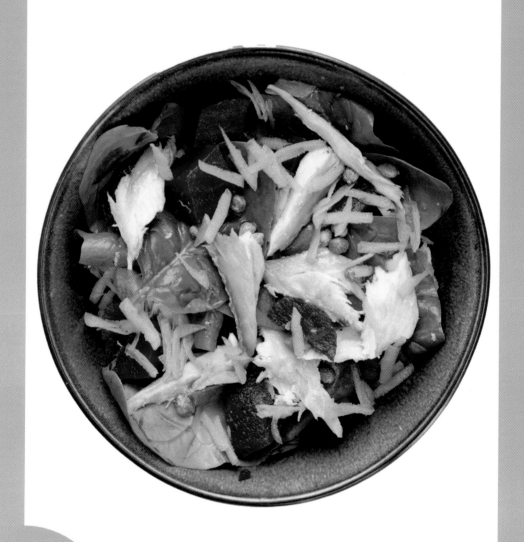

MACKEREL AND BEETROOT SALAD

As the mackerel is quite buttery and the beetroot moist, you don't miss having a dressing on this salad. The tang of the capers just makes it sing!

FACT SHEET

Serves 2

Prep time 5 minutes

Per portion 395 calories 34g protein 12g carbohydrate

INGREDIENTS

2 smoked mackerel fillets

2 small pre-cooked beetroot

4 handfuls of young spinach

1 tbsp of nonpareil capers

1 small carrot grated

Salt, black pepper and lemon juice to taste

METHOD

Remove skin from mackerel fillets and roughly break up.

Chop beetroot into 2cm chunks.

Put all ingredients into a bowl and lightly mix.

Add salt, pepper and lemon juice to taste and divide between two bowls.

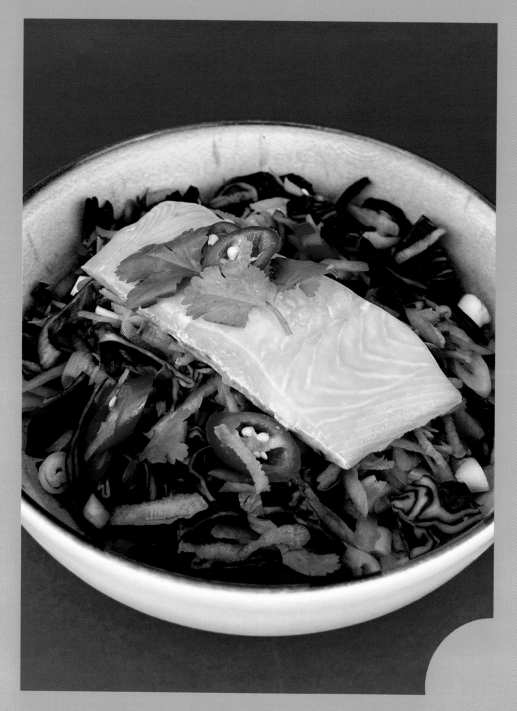

SALMON WITH ASIAN SLAW

For a speedy lunch I buy pre-cooked salmon fillets, but this also works with fresh salmon cooked in the oven in foil for 20 mins. Just add Thai green curry paste and a sprinkle of desiccated coconut before cooking.

If you want to take it to work with you, keep the dressing separate in a small container to keep the salad fresh and crunchy.

FACT SHEET

Serves 2

Prep time

Per portion 453 calories 41g protein 9g carbohydrate

INGREDIENTS

¼ of a small red cabbage finely chopped

1 carrot grated

4 spring onions chopped

2 red chillies chopped

Handful of coriander chopped (large or small depending on how much you like it)

1 tbsp sesame oil

1 tbsp rice vinegar

2 tbsp mirin

2 cooked salmon fillets

1 tbsp sesame seeds

Salt and pepper to taste

METHOD

Combine all the ingredients apart from salmon in a bowl and mix.

Divide between two bowls and place the salmon on top.

Garnish with more sesame seeds and season.

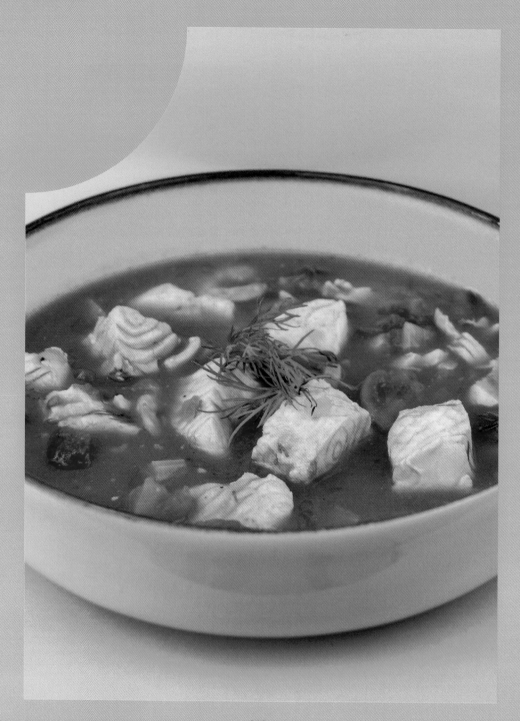

SEAFOOD SOUP

A quick, easy and filling take on bouillabaisse, which is easy as I always have fish in the fridge. Salmon is a great source of Omega 3, of which the benefits are multifold and covered in the next section.

FACT SHEET

Serves 2

Prep time

Cooking time

Per portion 343 calories 57g protein 16g carbohydrate

INGREDIENTS

200g salmon fillet skin off

150g cod loin

150g cooked large prawns

1 banana shallot

Extra virgin olive oil

Garlic paste

400g canned chopped tomatoes

2 star anise

Salt and pepper

Fish stock cube

200ml water

1 tbsp of fresh chopped dill

METHOD

Chop salmon and cod into 2.5 cm chunks.

Finely chop shallot.

Heat a large heavy bottomed pan with 2 tsp of olive oil.

Add the shallot and soften for about 5 mins till transparent.

Add garlic paste and stir for 1 minute.

Add tomatoes, water, stock cubes, star anise and bring to the boil.

Add the cod and salmon and then simmer for 8 minutes or till fish cooked.

Add fresh dill and prawns. Cook for 3–4 mins until prawns warmed through. Season as needed with salt and pepper.

Remove star anise and serve in warm bowls.

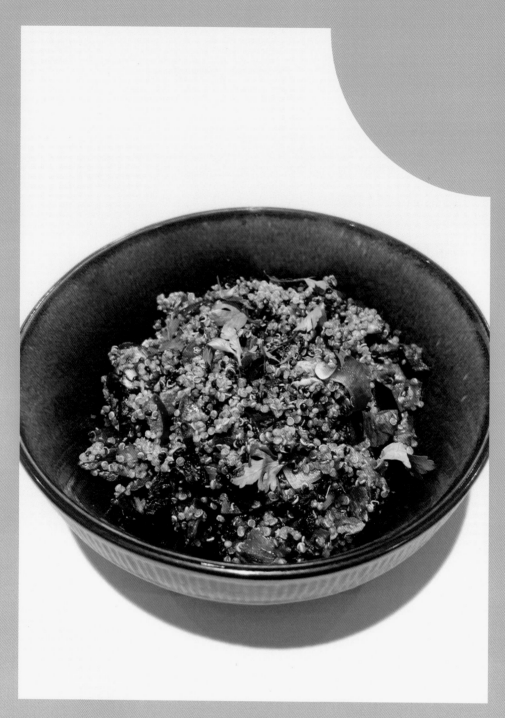

MUSHROOM "QUISSOTO"

Having found out that quinoa has more protein than rice (because it is a seed, not a grain), I wanted to experiment by adding it to one of my favourite dishes. This mushroom risotto with quinoa doesn't have the creaminess of traditional risotto but with the addition of dried porcini mushrooms there is still a rich, earthy taste. It's a lovely lunch, but also a great side for a main course of chicken or venison.

FACT SHEET

Serves 2

Prep time 25 mins

Cooking time 10 mins

Per portion 335 calories 9g protein 38g carbohydrate

INGREDIENTS

30g dried porcini mushrooms

1/2 red onion

Spray olive oil

100g chestnut mushrooms

50ml boiling water

1 250gm packet of pre-cooked red and white quinoa

Dried thyme

1 tsp mirin

Salt and pepper

METHOD

In a small dish, add the dried porcini mushrooms to boiled water. Allow to soak for 20 mins while you prepare the rest of the recipe.

Finely chop the red onion.

Add spray oil to a medium pan and warm to a medium heat. Add chopped onions and soften for about 10 mins till transparent.

While it's softening, finely slice the chestnut mushrooms then add to the pan with the thyme, stirring for about 6–8 mins while they soften.

When the porcini has soaked for 20 mins take out and finely chop saving the water.

Add the chopped porcini, the mirin, the soaking water and the quinoa to the pan and thoroughly heat through allowing the porcini flavours to merge with the other ingredients. After a couple of minutes serve up in bowls.

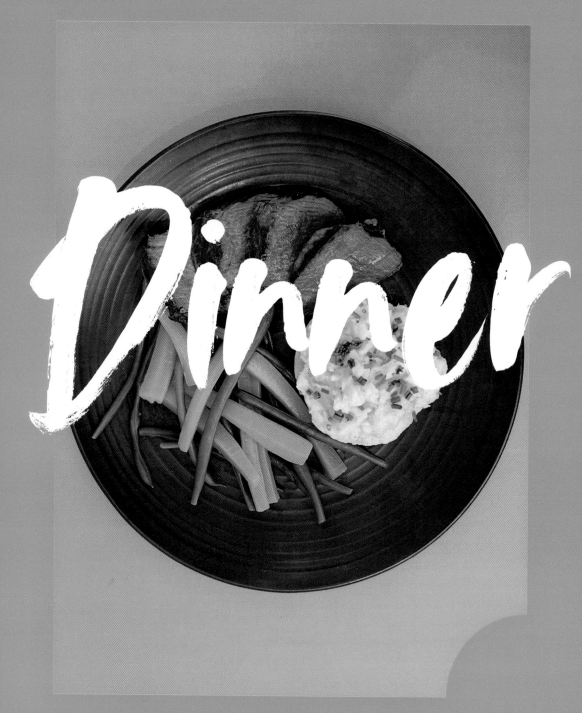

Dinner

GRILLED VENISON STEAK WITH CELERIAC

I have always enjoyed a good, grass-fed fillet steak, cooked rare.

When I had to make heathy swaps, I learned that venison has around half the calories and a sixth of the saturated fat of beef, with more protein, vitamins, and minerals.

Celeriac has less than half the carbohydrate and calories of potatoes and can be eaten raw or cooked. I serve this with instant gravy (I told you I was a quick cook) but if you want to make a fancy sauce, over to you.

FACT SHEET

Prep time 5 mins

Cooking time 25 mins

Per portion 236 calories 50g protein 9g carbohydrate

INGREDIENTS

400g venison loin

Glug of extra virgin olive oil

400g celeriac chopped into 2.5cm cubes.

160g green beans

1 tbsp of chopped chives

Salt and pepper

METHOD

Preheat oven to 200 degrees or 180 degrees for fan oven.

Season the venison loin with salt.

Heat a heavy bottomed frying pan, ideally one that can go into the oven and add olive oil.

When hot, sear the venison loin on all sides.

Whilst this is happening, put celeriac cubes in a saucepan and cover with water. Bring to the boil and simmer for 15 mins.

When venison is cooked on all sides, and while celeriac cooks, put the pan into oven (or put in pre-warmed metal tray) for 10 mins. The venison should still be slightly pink in the middle.

Take the meat out as it will need to rest for 5–10 mins to avoid leaking the juices into your mash.

Heat a small pan of boiling water for the beans which will take 6–7 mins while venison rests.

Now is the time to drain and mash the celeriac, adding seasoning.

When everything is ready, slice up the venison into thick chunks, pile up the mash and garnish with chives before serving alongside the beans.

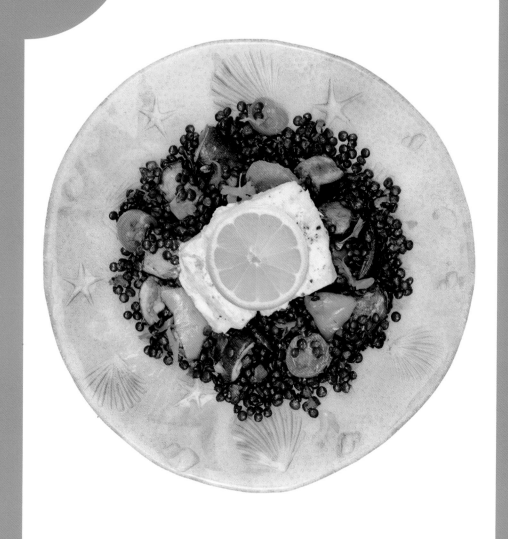

COD LOIN WITH ROASTED MEDITERRANEAN VEGETABLES AND PUY LENTILS

Lentils became one of the substitutes for rice, pasta or potato, as they are very high source of protein. My quick hack is to use pre-cooked ones then add different ingredients.

FACT SHEET

Serves 2

Prep time 10 mins

Cooking time 40 mins

Per portion 485 calories 49g Protein 30g carbohydrate

INGREDIENTS

1 small yellow pepper

1 small courgette

½ red onion

½ large aubergine

Spray olive oil

2 cod loins 200gm each

1 250g packet of pre-cooked puy/ green lentils

Handful fresh flat leaf parsley chopped

1 lemon

METHOD

Preheat oven to 200 degrees or 180 degrees for fan oven.

Chop pepper, courgette and aubergine into 2cm chunks.

Put into a metal baking dish, spray with olive oil and put into the oven for 40 mins.

Prepare some foil big enough to wrap the cod in. Place the two loins in the middle and season with salt and pepper. Lay a thick slice of lemon on each. Wrap the foil around to make a parcel then place on baking sheet.

With 20 mins to go, put the cod into the oven.

With 5 mins left on the timer, heat the lentils as instructed on packet.

When vegetables are cooked, tip the warmed lentils and chopped parsley into the baking dish, squeeze in extra lemon juice and seasoning and mix

Serve up the lentils onto warm plates then remove cod from foil and place on top.

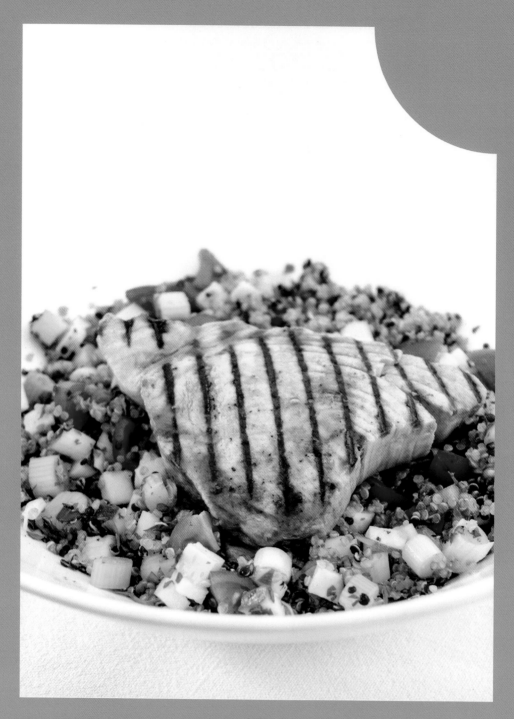

SEARED TUNA WITH HERBY QUINOA

FACT SHEET

Serves 2

Prep time 10 mins

Cooking time 10-15 mins

Per portion 453 calories Protein 58g Carbohydrate 39g

INGREDIENTS

2 tuna steaks

2 tbsp lime juice

2 tbsp of light soy sauce

1 250g packet ready cooked red and white quinoa

3 spring onions

Small bunch of flat leaf parsley

Small bunch of mint

½ courgette

6 cherry tomatoes

Salt and black pepper

Spray olive oil

Dried chilli flakes

METHOD

In a bowl big enough to hold tuna steaks put in soy sauce, 1 tbsp of lime juice and salt and pepper. Stir and add tuna steaks to the marinade whilst you prepare the quinoa. Chop the spring onions, the tomatoes and the courgette into small, evenly sized pieces (around 1cm). Finely chop the parsley and mint.

Add these ingredients to the packet of quinoa with second tbsp of lime juice and mix well.

Heat a frying pan with the olive oil, on a fairly high heat, then cook tuna for 2-3 mins each side if you like pink in the middle or 4 mins if you like cooked through. You may need to vary this depending on thickness of the steak.

When cooked, divide the quinoa between two plates and serve the tuna on top, sprinkled with some chilli flakes to taste.

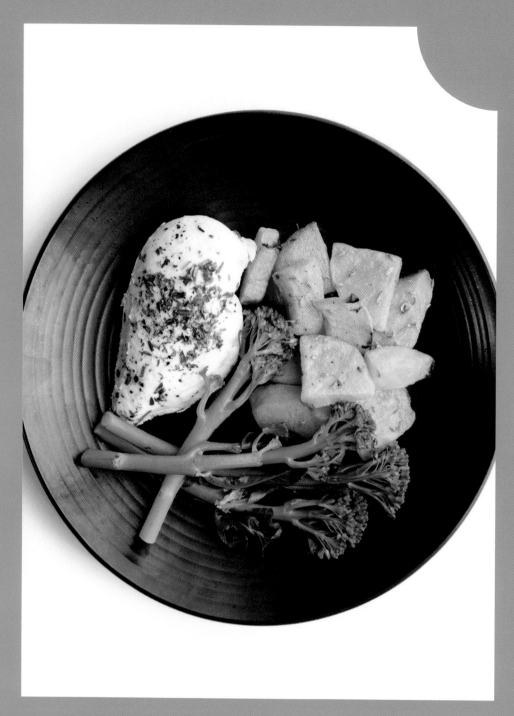

ROAST CHICKEN WITH ROASTED SQUASH AND BROCCOLI

FACT SHEET

Serves 2

Prep time 5 mins

Cooking time 40 minutes

Per portion 378 calories 44g Protein 44g carbohydrate

INGREDIENTS

300g of butternut squash chopped into 3cm chunks

2 chicken breast fillets

8 stems of long stem broccoli (or more if you love it)

Salt and pepper

1–2 tsp dried tarragon

1 dessert spoon fennel seeds

Spray olive oil

METHOD

Preheat oven to 200 degrees or 180 degrees for fan oven.

Arrange butternut squash on a baking tray and spray with 3–4 squirts of olive oil.

Sprinkle over fennel seeds and put into top of oven for 40 mins.

Get a piece of foil large enough to wrap both chicken breasts.

Place chicken in centre of the foil and add salt, pepper and sprinkle over tarragon. Wrap foil around the chicken and seal.

Put on a baking tray and put in the oven when squash has 20 mins to go.

Fill a medium pan with water and bring to the boil. Add broccoli and cook for 7 mins.

When all items are ready plate up and drizzle with extra virgin olive oil if you like or add a chicken gravy.

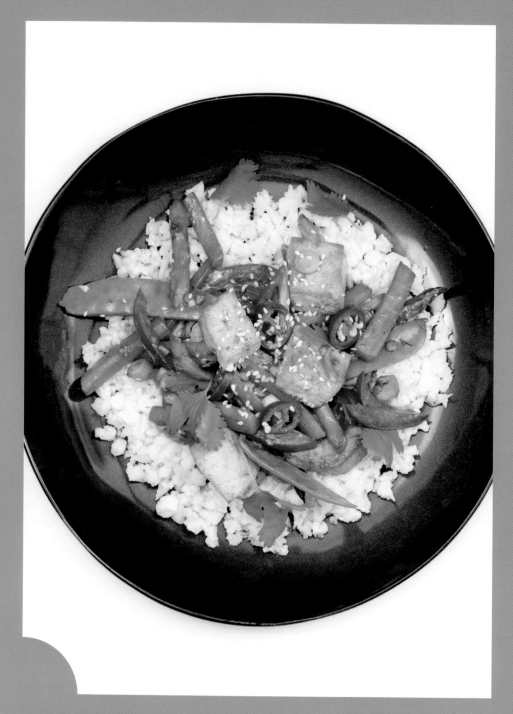

STIR-FRIED TOFU AND VEGETABLES WITH CAULIFLOWER RICE

FACT SHEET

Serves 2

Prep time 10 mins

Cooking time 20 mins

INGREDIENTS

200g cauliflower florets

400g smoked organic tofu

Sesame seed oil

1 small carrot

1 small red pepper

4 asparagus spears

Large handful of mangetout

1 fresh red chilli

Handful fresh coriander

2 dessert spoons of crunchy peanut butter

2 tbsp soy sauce

150ml water

Sesame seeds

METHOD

Start with preparing your cauliflower rice by finely chopping your florets into small rice size pieces.

Next, take the tofu and cut into 2–2.5cm chunks.

Heat some oil in a large frying pan to a fairly high heat and brown off tofu on all sides, this will take about 6 mins. Set aside while you cook the vegetables.

Slice the pepper and carrots into slim batons and the asparagus into similar lengths 4–5cm.

Heat the large frying pan again then add the vegetables stirring for 6–8 minutes until they start to soften slightly.

Add the tofu to the pan with the peanut butter, water and soy sauce and throw in the mangetout (add water to make the sauce the right consistency for you).

Pop the cauliflower rice into the microwave in a bowl with a cover for 2 ½ minutes 850 or 2 minutes on 1000.

When cooked, put onto a plate with a well for the stir fry.

Just before serving the stir-fry on top, add chopped coriander and chopped red chilli.

To finish off sprinkle with sesame seeds.

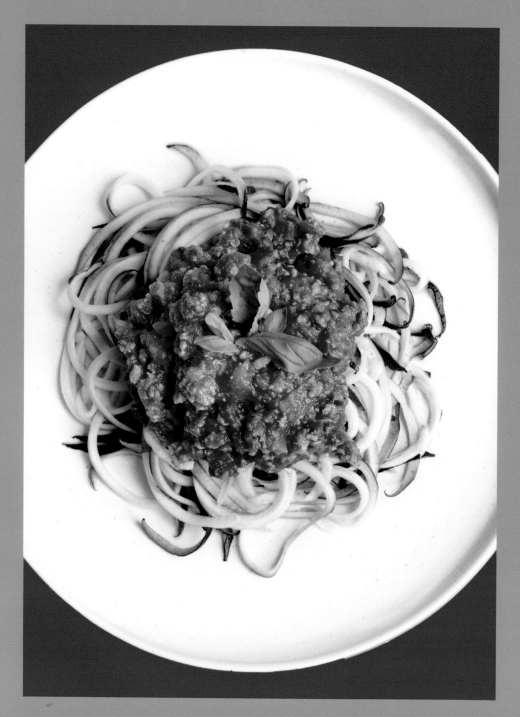

TURKEY BOLOGNESE WITH COURGETTI

FACT SHEET

Serves 2

Prep time 10 mins

Cooking time 25 minutes

Per portion 397 calories 20g Protein 11g carbohydrate

INGREDIENTS

1 small red onion

2 rashers of fat free bacon

400g tin of chopped tomatoes

250g of 2% turkey mince

1 tbsp of tomato puree

1/4 tsp of truvia

2 sticks of celery

1 chicken stock cube/pot

1 large courgette

2 tsp dried oregano

2 tsp dried or handful of fresh chopped basil

Spray olive oil

Salt and pepper

METHOD

Finely chop up the bacon, celery and red onion.

Heat some oil in a large frying pan to a medium heat and the vegetables and cook for 5–6 mins until onion starts to go transparent.

Add the chopped bacon and stir for another 5 mins.

Add the turkey mince and brown, breaking it up so there are no lumps about 5 mins.

When browned add the chopped tomato, truvia, stock and dried herbs (if using fresh basil, I add at the end).

Bring to the boil then simmer for 15 mins.

Spiralise the courgette (I have a simple hand spiraliser).

4 mins before the sauce is ready, put the courgetti in a microwaveable bowl, cover with film and pierce.

Cook for 3 mins on full power. Drain any liquid off. Divide between serving plates.

Serve the bolognese sauce piled on top of the courgetti adding fresh basil on top if desired.

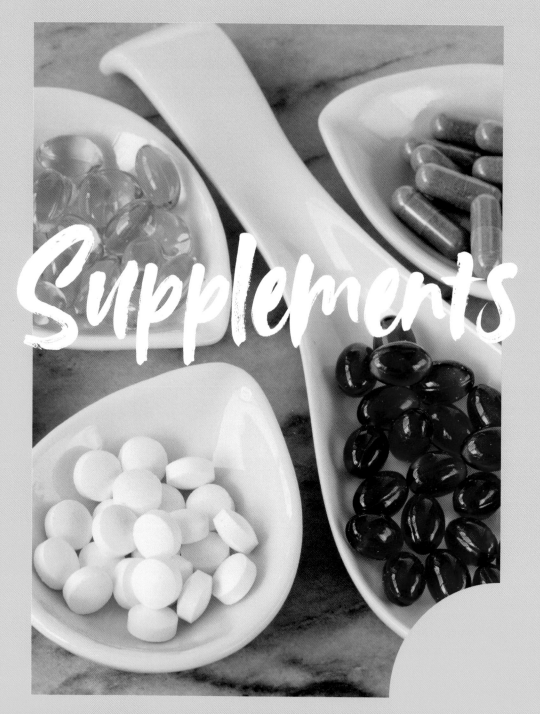

Supplements

The world of supplements is vast. It can be overwhelming when trying to work out the good from the bad.

Here, I will tell you what I take, and why. After reading up on the benefits and trying various supplements, these are ones I noticed that made, and still make a positive difference in my body.

GLUCOSAMINE AND CHONDROITIN

With arthritis in the family and creaky knees from running, for me these are an aid and a preventative. These natural compounds, are neither vitamins or minerals but they offer incredible benefits. Glucosamine and Chondroitin are the regular pairing for joint health. Together they support cartilage health and reduce joint discomfort, maintaining my flexibility and mobility.

Cartilage Protection

These compounds work in a complementary way to promote the strength and flexibility of cartilage, crucial for my active lifestyle.

Anti-Inflammatory

They are a natural anti-inflammatory, giving relief from joint inflammation and stiffness and helping me stay agile.

Improved Joint Function

They help joint function by maintaining and lubricating the joints, helping smoother movement and reduced friction. They help with recovery after exercise or physical activities. Glucosamine and Chondroitin assist in supporting the repair process of joints and connective tissues.

COLLAGEN

I initially started taking this as its marketing heavily implied that it plumped up your skin; and with the natural changes that occur in your skin as you get older, I fancied that. I have subsequently learnt that there are so many more benefits.

Glowing Skin

Collagen is the building block of our skin, maintaining its elasticity, firmness, and hydration. I definitely noticed a more radiant, youthful glow!

Joint Health

Enhance joint flexibility and mobility. Collagen supports the tendons and ligaments, aiding in reducing joint discomfort and supporting an active lifestyle. I definitely need that.

Hair & Nail Strength

With fine hair that was also thinning with hormonal changes, I found that this helped massively. Collagen strengthens hair and nails and encourages growth. Although I certainly don't have long flowing hair, I think it's one of the things that has stopped my hair and nails from being so fragile.

Gut Health

It supports your digestive system. Collagen assists in maintaining the integrity of the gut lining, promoting a healthy digestive tract.

Muscle Mass

With an increase in weight bearing exercise in the mix of what I do, I have looked to supplements that aid muscle repair and growth. Collagen plays a crucial role in supporting muscle strength and recovery.

L-CARNITINE

I hadn't heard of this, but as I started to study personal training, and learned of the benefits, I thought it could help me. I saw my body change with more muscle definition as I started to take it.

Energy Ignition

L-Carnitine is your metabolism's best friend, aiding in the conversion of fat into energy. It maximises the impact of your workouts. Its main role in your body involves mitochondrial function and energy production. It helps to transport fatty acids into the mitochondria. Mitochondria are the cells which generate most of the chemical energy to fire up muscles and nerve cells as well as many other functions. They are the energy convertors. I have read it can improve high intensity exercise performance when taken 60–90 minutes before working out so I have it first thing in the morning with my other supplements.

Fat Loss Support

It enhances the body's fat-burning capacity. As seen above, L-Carnitine helps transport fatty acids to the mitochondria for fuel, contributing to a leaner you. Due to this, it's sometimes used as a weight loss supplement.

Muscle Recovery

It supports post-workout recovery. L-Carnitine aids in reducing muscle soreness and fatigue, promoting faster recuperation. It is commonly added to sports supplements due to its rapid absorption rate. It may aid muscle soreness and recovery in exercise.

Cardiovascular Health

L-Carnitine plays a role in reducing oxidative stress, supporting a healthy heart and circulation. They help produce the iron compound needed to transport oxygen. In studies it was found that L-carnitine significantly reduced diastolic blood pressure, especially in people who were overweight and obese.

MAGNESIUM

From thorough research, I have learned that magnesium is an essential mineral that plays a crucial role in various physiological functions within the body. It can be found in magnesium-rich foods such as nuts, seeds, leafy green vegetables, and whole grains but if you don't get enough through diet, can be taken as a supplement.

Muscle Function and Relaxation

Magnesium is vital for muscle function and is often used to help prevent muscle cramps and spasms. It works together with calcium to regulate muscle contractions and promote overall muscle relaxation. As I have gained years, I seem to get cramp more often, and I find that this really helps.

Healthy Bones

Magnesium contributes to bone health by working with calcium and vitamin D to help build and maintain strong bones. It is estimated that about 60% of magnesium in the body is actually found in bones. Studies link increased magnesium intake with increased overall bone mineral density.

More Energy

Magnesium is involved in the production and transfer of energy within cells, which helps with your workouts. It plays a critical role in the synthesis of adenosine triphosphate (ATP), which is what fires up muscle cells.

Calms the nervous system

Magnesium is known to help reduce stress and anxiety. It regulates neurotransmitters, which are important for mood and overall mental well-being.

Heart Health

Magnesium supports heart health by helping regulate blood pressure and maintaining a regular heartbeat. It also plays a role in the relaxation of blood vessels. Magnesium may help protect heart health by reducing inflammation and maintaining the function of the cell membranes.

Aids Sleep

Magnesium is often most associated with improving sleep quality. It helps relax muscles and has a calming effect on the nervous system, promoting better sleep. It's not completely clear how it works, researchers believe that magnesium deficiency could alter the sleep-wake cycle, leading to symptoms of insomnia.

Digestive Health

Magnesium can help regulate bowel movements and has a mild laxative effect (anyone remember Milk of Magnesia being given?). It can be used to relieve constipation, something that is often aggravated with hormonal changes.

Blood Sugar Regulation

Magnesium is involved in insulin function and the regulation of blood sugar levels. Adequate magnesium levels may contribute to a reduced risk of type 2 diabetes.

Research shows it could play a part in regulating insulin; the hormone responsible for transporting sugar from the bloodstream to the cells.

HYALURONIC ACID

I have used this externally as a serum for my skin, but I also now take it as a supplement, having learned more about its benefits. It is a chain like molecule called a polymer which binds water and other molecules through the body. It's found in bone broth, oranges, tofu, kale, almonds, edamame, and sweet potato.

Healthier Plumped Skin

Used as a serum or as a supplement, hyaluronic acid can improve overall skin health. It improves its elasticity, increases skin moisture and makes it more supple and soft. By the nature of doing this it softens wrinkles making your face appear smoother. I noticed a visible difference once I started.

Helps Wounds Heal

Its chain like structure means it acts like a scaffold for tissue to grow which is a key part to the body healing wounds including muscle repair or minor scarring. It regulates inflammation levels and has been shown to decrease pain faster. It also has anti-bacterial properties.

Joint Health

Hyaluronic acid is naturally found in joints to keep them lubricated. With better lubrication the bones are less likely to grind against each other so it's very helpful for easing osteo arthritis.

Helps Dry Eyes

One of the symptoms of peri-menopause and menopause is dry eyes. Hyaluronic eye drops reduce symptoms. While it's not clear at the moment if oral supplements help, as I take them anyway it could be an added benefit.

OMEGA 3

I originally started to take Cod Liver Oil capsules for my aching knee joints. The main component in cod liver oil is Omega 3, which not only reduces inflammation, it supports heart health and boosts brain function. However, a note of caution here; it is essential to make sure that there are also fat-soluble polyphenols in it to support it reaching the cellular level. Polyphenols are the game-changer with any fish oil supplement as they chaperone Omega 3, ensuring it reaches its destination intact.

The best source of Omega 3 is in fatty fish such as wild salmon (not farmed, as industrial fish feed may be high in in Omega 6 which is pro-inflammatory), mackerel, herring, tuna, sardines, pilchards, oyster, crab, shrimp. A 1000 mg a day is recommended. Omega 3 is also available in foods such as walnuts almonds, chia seeds, flax and hemp seeds. A more useful alternative for vegetarians and vegans for instance would be to take a marine algal oil, which contains exactly the same omega 3's as occur in fish oil and which the body can use directly.
Source:
Let Your Food Be Your Pharmaco-Nutrition Dr. Paul Clayton

Alternatively, there are also lots of foods to enjoy rich in polyphenols to support the Omega 3 journey, which are also anti-inflammatory, good for your heart and improve insulin sensitivity decreasing the risk of diabetes. Found in berries, cocoa (hello, dark chocolate!) spices, nuts, seeds, red wine, olives and olive oil all of which I love.

Joint Support

Cod liver oil's anti-inflammatory properties may help in reducing joint pain and stiffness. They have anti-inflammatory properties and as my father has debilitating arthritis, I am a fan, as it can suppress the symptoms of prolonged inflammatory diseases like arthritis.

Vitamin D Boost

This is the sunshine vitamin. Cod liver oil is a fantastic source of vitamin D, crucial for strong bones and a robust immune system.

Radiant Skin

Achieve a healthy glow as the omega-3s and vitamins in cod liver oil promote radiant skin.

You should start to see the difference when taking it after 3 months. It helps regulate oil production, improve hydration and minimises signs of aging. It can have a soothing effect on dermatitis and irritated skin.

Weight loss

Omega 3 in cod liver oil with polyphenols may help you lose inches and shed body fat. It can be useful for decreasing appetite if you're on a weight loss diet. This is because ingesting fish oil containing polyphenols can helps your body to switch from using carbs to fats as a source of fuel during exercise.

Mood Uplifter

Beat the blues naturally. The fatty acids in cod liver oil are linked to mood regulation, helping you to stay positive and energized. They combat psychological conditions such as depression and schizophrenia.

With the right diet choices, you may not need all these supplements, as I explained these are my choices for my concerns. Remember, quality matters. Look for a reputable source to ensure you're getting all the fantastic benefits without compromise. I am going to continue to learn more about nutrition and supplements for the body as I have found that they can have a huge impact on your quality of life.

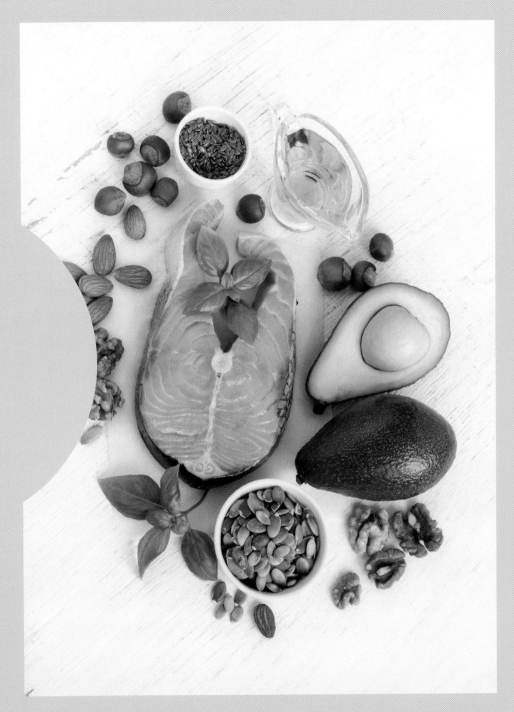

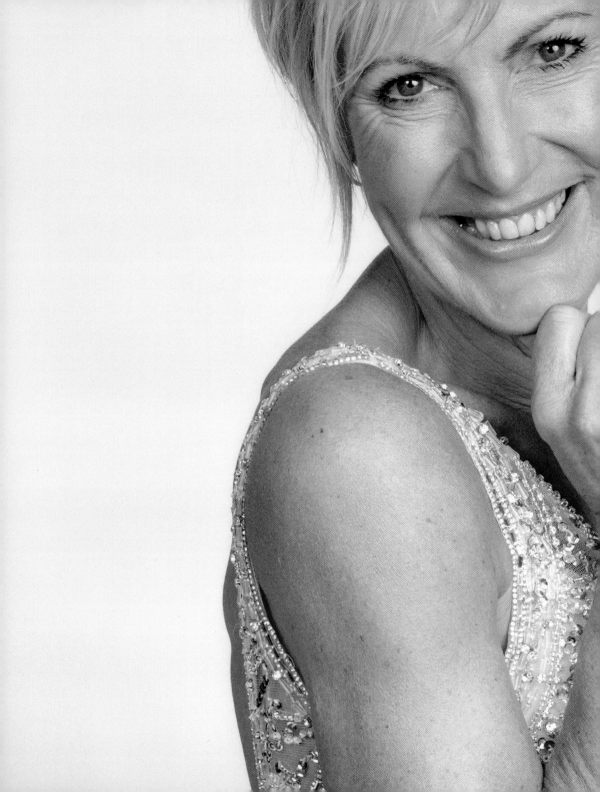

CHAPTER 11

STYLE FOR THE NEW YOU

STYLE IS KNOWING WHAT SUITS YOU

As Coco Chanel famously said, "Fashion fades where style remains."

I've always believed that style is not defined by the latest trends, but by the confidence you exude when you wear what makes you feel your best.

Fashion is your own personal canvas and you can make it a masterpiece!

Let your style reflect your personality, your creativity and your inner sparkle. Fashion is a powerful tool that can lift your spirits, boost confidence and let you shine in your own unique way. When you put on an outfit that makes you feel unstoppable, you strut your stuff with confidence. From casual chic to red carpet glam, I'm all about embracing different styles.

Most importantly, remember that you absolutely don't have to dress your age! If you have fabulous legs and want to wear a mini skirt, do it. If you have great shoulders, show them off.

One thing to look out for if your body shape has changed; don't dress in clothes that suited the old you. You will look and feel different after the 90 days. It may be that you now have more body confidence, so this is the perfect time to experiment. If before you hid under clothes, you might be surprised about what suits you now. Go shopping with your best cheerleader friend (but one who will also be honest with you if things don't suit you) and make a day of it. But remember…

QUALITY BEATS QUANTITY

If you need to invest in some new pieces now that you have changed shape or size, this is the time to do it.

My advice is to buy less, but buy better. You will really treasure these pieces as you worked hard for them.

With some high quality, versatile staples that you can style up or down, you are supporting the need for sustainability in the fashion industry and won't regret the investment. Buy now, wear forever.

THINGS I HAVE BEEN ABLE TO RE-WEAR FOR YEARS...

TEA-DRESS

One of the first big successes in my career came when I designed an incredibly popular navy dot-print tea-dress for Next. It was a classic-fit flared button through number with a shirred, elastic section at the waist. If it was in the store today you wouldn't blink twice as these days the shape appears in everyone's collections because it's just so flattering. If you buy a print you love, rather than one that's fashionable at the time, it will reflect your personality and you will always feel good in it. I have a vintage Vivienne Westwood one, a huge inspiration to me as a designer. The print is based on Mattise, my favourite artist, and it fills me with joy to wear it. A tea

dress works layered with knits, blazers and coats, with trainers, heels or boots. You can even layer it over a...

BLACK MERINO ROLL NECK

Simple and elegant, a fine knitted roll neck will complement almost any shape. If you want a sophisticated office look, you can wear with tailored trousers. I particularly like the slim roll neck shape with a wide leg pant, 1940's style. Think how great old Hollywood film stars like Lauren Bacall looked or how this silhouette is always on the catwalks. If they are high waisted, even better. They can make your legs look like they go on forever. Layer with a structured blazer or toughen up with a biker jacket.

A black roll neck is also the perfect base to add a statement skirt. I have a few of these in my wardrobe. Whether a maxi tulle skirt, a bold coloured knee length satin or a tailored leather skirt, the polo is the best support act.

A roll neck sweater of course works equally well with high-waisted jeans or skinny jeans. Untucked, it gives a relaxed look which I particularly like beneath a blazer.

Merino is a lovely, soft fibre to wear that regulates your body temperature. It keeps you cool when its warm or warms you up when it's cool and naturally wicks moisture away from the body and is often used for ski base layers (that's why Merino sheep wear it!). It's renewable and sustainable and if looked after with careful washing, will stay looking gorgeous for a long time.

CLASSIC MAC

You can't beat a timeless trench coat in a neutral colour like beige or camel (think Burberry). It's perfect for both rainy days and adds sophistication to any outfit. This style works just as well over a knee length dress or with trousers. Depending on the look, you can cinch at the waist or knot the belt behind for a swing shape. I have a vintage Burberry mac in heavy black lace which I love as a twist on the classic. It still doesn't date but always makes a statement. They may not be as waterproof as some hi-tech options, but I have an umbrella. I also found in the back of a wardrobe an old 1980's mac of my mums, with big shoulders and a button out check inner liner which I love. Both proof that this piece stands the test of time.

JEANS

These are hard to narrow down. I have three shapes that have stood the test of time.

First there's the wide leg in dark denim, with a faint pinstripe which always look great with just a simple white tee in summer or a slim knit in winter. This style works best with a flat shoe, a trainer or a lace up flat boot. A crop, culotte version works too. If you are petite, you may find that this style suits you better.

Next, I have to mention the stretch skinny. Yes, they may officially come and go with fashion trends, but as we wear what suits us now, we don't care. If you like a baggier top, whether it's a big loose knit or shirt, the slim shape balances this out. I like them with ankle boots, riding boots or trainers. With a heel they can be worn with a sparkly top from pub to club.

Finally, there is the washed boyfriend jean. This is the weekend casual go-to. It needs to be in super soft laundered denim so that it is relaxed around your curves and not too tight, perfect for that just-borrowed look. If they are in a mid to light colour, they could be a year old or 20 years old. No-one will know, they will just want to get the look!

OVERSIZED CASHMERE V-NECK

A quality cashmere sweater in a neutral tone like grey, navy, or camel will never date. I confess to also owning them in bright pink and cobalt blue, as they are my colours. I personally like a v-neck as it elongates the neck and makes your shoulders look narrower versus a crew, which can make you look wider. It's cosy, versatile and perfect for layering during cooler months or for travelling on planes when you need something that's not too bulky but warm enough for when the air-conditioning sets in.

I have lost a couple of my favourite jumpers to moths, so now put them in the freezer to kill any eggs before packing away for summer in a zip lock plastic bag. I also learned how to darn holes in knitwear when I studied needlework at school. I think it's a long-lost art that should be revived.

WRAP WOOL COAT

Having worked as Managing Director for Jaeger, I can vouch for the durability of this classic style. The camel hair fabric was an invention of Jaeger and with it, the classic camel coat was born. A mid-calf length will work with most outfits, there will be a tone of camel that is right for your skin whether it's a blonde, lighter tone or a darker vicuna level.

LBD (LITTLE BLACK DRESS)

A versatile, well-fitted black dress that can be dressed up or down for different events, from formal occasions to casual outings, is a must have. If you find a shape that suits you, hang on to it. I like a sleeveless, tailored shift as it works under a blazer and can be worn as an evening cocktail dress with heels and a statement necklace. Equally, they can be layered over a roll neck or chiffon blouse to get a completely different look.

An LBJ (Little Black Jumpsuit) should be on the list too, as the all-in-one silhouette is flatteringly elongating. A tailored shape will give you an hourglass figure.

BLACK TROUSERS

All of us will have some black trousers in the wardrobe. There are two shapes I have worn on repeat over the years. One is a wide leg, with a flat brogue shoe and a narrower-cut top to balance out the wide leg. The other is a slim 7/8th length, or ankle grazer, with a larger looser sweater or shirt. They can take a trainer, a ballet flat, a loafer or a heel, so make a fabulous multitasker.

If you go for a good quality fabric, ideally with a little stretch in it, and you look after them, they will last. Never iron on the right side as the fabric may shine.

BLACK RIDING BOOTS

I have a pair of beautiful black leather riding boots I bought in Barneys in NY in 2001. I have had them re-soled 3 times (worth doing) but the boot leather has remained perfect. There's something very rewarding about polishing them and knowing that the shoe polish nourished them and keeps them supple, a bit like moisturiser. I find it quite sad that shoe polish manufacturers like Kiwi stopped selling polish in the UK as no-one polishes their shoes anymore, buying more cheap imitation leather and throwing them away. Through the years I've worn them with skinny jeans, floaty dresses, black miniskirts and opaque tights, as well as jeans and jumpers. They were expensive at the time but the cost per wear is now very low and I will continue to cherish them.

VINTAGE SILK SCARF

I started collecting these in the '80s. They can add personality and pizzazz to an outfit. They can be worn around the neck and tied so many different ways. They can also be tied to a handbag, worn as a headband on a bad hair day and used as a tie belt with jeans to add a splash of colour. I have even knotted two together to make a halter neck or bandeau top.

MANNISH BUTTON-UP SHIRT

A crisp, white or classic blue and white stripe button-up shirt is a wardrobe staple. Go for a good quality 100% cotton option and it will improve with age. I like to style these in various ways; they are great with jeans at weekends, can be layered under a jumper or thrown on as a beach cover up. A mannish shirt can also be worn knotted at the waist or loose – so versatile!

WHITE LINEN KAFTAN

Linen is the perfect fabric for summer as it quickly absorbs moisture from the body then releases it into the air, which is why it's favoured in warm countries. A fresh, white kaftan is timeless. With Islamic origins, they were first seen in Europe in the 1890's when Queen Victoria's daughter stepped out in one. Yet they really grew in popularity in the 1920's when the designer Paul Poiret, who, inspired by the Ballet Russes, featured it in many of his designs (he's one of my favourite designers in the history of fashion). Since the boho look has now become a summer stalwart, you can't go wrong with this as a warm-weather blouse or swim cover-up.

TAILORED BLAZER

A well-cut blazer in a neutral colour like black or navy can elevate any outfit. Whether paired with jeans for a casual look or worn over a dress, a fine wool blend should not crease and will be light and comfortable. If your style is more casual or androgynous, you might like a looser cut. If you like a more feminine, curvy look, a tailored shape will be for you. I like a contrast lining in the sleeve as when rolled and pushed up they can lend a flash of colour. A quick style tip; elastic bands can hold rolled up sleeves in place and will remain hidden in the folds.

I also have an extensive button collection that I have accumulated over the years and you can easily switch up the look of a blazer by swapping plain dark buttons for gold or brushed silver.

WHITE TRAINERS OR LACE UP PUMPS

A pair of clean white trainers or pumps can be paired with jeans or printed dresses and can even make a tailored suit look cool. Find a pair you can stick in the washing machine to keep that box-fresh look and replace the laces if they get grubby. If you have these, they can all be versatile and changed or updated with accessories.

GREAT ACCESSORIES CAN MAKE AN OUTFIT

I remember as a young buyer observing my boss, who always looked incredible but only ever seemed to wear a uniform of dark trousers and simple tops. I realised that the source of her style was that she invested in stunning statement belts or jewellery and they elevated every outfit. If you choose items that call to you and reflect your style, they can say as much about you as any garment and make you feel like you own the room. I have a love of wings in jewellery and some fabulous pieces that I have owned for 20 years or more can still transform my outfit and draw comments at the supermarket checkout!

COLOUR IS GOOD FOR YOU

Life is too short to wear boring clothes! Style is not just about the clothes we wear; it's a form of self-expression, a way to tell the world who we are without saying a word.

The colours you wear say a lot about you. They can also influence how you feel.

Red – This is the colour of confidence and passion, so great for a first date or work presentation. I love red. I invested in a stunning red Alexander McQueen dress that caught my eye and I waited, crossing my fingers that it would end up in the sale. It did. It was one of the dresses I wore for my 60th birthday photo shoot and whenever I step into it, I step into confidence.

Yellow – The colour of sunshine generates happiness and uplifts us. As a blonde, I am very careful which shade of yellow I wear, but with a tan, a gorgeous egg yolk yellow works well for me. Be sure to experiment with the right shades for your skin tone and hair colour.

Blue – From calming softer blues to smarter navy, the qualities of this colour can be harnessed in several ways.

Pink – Make a positive, feminine statement with pink. I prefer stronger pinks with my slightly olive skin undertone but you might find pastel is more for you if you have more of a blush undertone.

Green – the colour for growth or feeling at one with nature. I have greens from verdant emerald to jewel-like teal in my wardrobe and always feel optimistic whenever I wear them.

There is always room for black and grey in your wardrobe, but with colouring changing as we mature, live life a little more boldly! Not only will it suit you but it can make you feel amazing too.

DRESSING FOR YOUR BODY SHAPE: CONFIDENCE IS KEY

Ultimately, you should wear what makes you feel confident and comfortable. Embrace your body shape and celebrate your best features. Here are some tips…

PETITE

- One colour or tonal dressing is a good way to look taller as it lengthens the body, rather than cutting you in half.

- Tailored pieces that fit properly. This includes trousers, skirts, and dresses that are proportionate to your frame. Alter where needed as excess material won't celebrate your petite stature.

- High-Waisted trousers, skirts, or shorts visually lengthen the legs and create the illusion of height. Wear with crop tops or tucked in shirts and it will highlight your waist.

- V-necks and vertical details like button or zip through tops and dresses draw the eye upward. The detail creates a vertical line that can make you appear taller. This elongates the neckline and lengthens the body.

- Heels or pointed-toe shoes and boots can add height and lengthen the legs. If you wear nude coloured ones when wearing skin tone hosiery and dresses, or black boots with black trousers, it creates a sleeker look. Avoid shoes with ankle straps that can visually shorten the legs.

- Shift dresses that finish on or above the knee will make your legs look longer than below the knee. Alternatively, opt for maxi skirts or dresses with high slits to create the illusion of longer legs while showing some skin for an elongated look.

BIGGER-BUSTED

- Start with a well-fitted, supportive bra that provides proper lift and ensures comfort. It is definitely worth getting re-measured for the correct fit if your body shape has changed, rather than guessing the new size required. A good bra will improve your posture and make clothing fit better.

- V-necklines are my preferred neckline as they draw attention upward and create a flattering silhouette. They elongate the neckline and can help balance out the bust with the rest of the body.

- Wrap dresses and tops can be very flattering for larger busts as they accentuate the waist, providing just the right amount of coverage and support if you are proud of your cleavage.

- Avoid high necklines as these emphasise the bust too much and can make it look larger. Opt for open necklines instead.

- Layer with well-cut tailoring, structured blazers and jackets. Waistcoats can add structure that complements the curves and balances out proportions.

- Embrace the waist! Clothing that cinches at the waist like belted dresses or tops create an hourglass shape to be proud of.

- Avoid empire line or smock shapes as they will flare out from the widest part of your body, making you look larger overall. Instead, try gentle swing shapes or blouson dresses which gather at the waist.

- Adjustable straps and necklines can be lowered or raised to suit your size and shape.

PEAR SHAPE

- A curvy bottom is celebrated now, so depending on how you feel you can choose what to wear.

- Highlighting the upper body with detailing around the neckline, like boat necks, square necks, or embellished tops will draw attention upwards. Statement sleeves, ruffles or bold patterns on blouses can emphasise the shoulders and bust, balancing out your overall shape.

- A-Line and fit-and-flare dresses that flare out from the waist can minimise focus on the hips and accentuate the waist beautifully.

- Bodycon dresses will celebrate your curves if you love your bum.

- High-waisted skirts or pants that cinch at the natural waist accentuate the slimmest part of the body. Wide-leg trousers or bootcut pants balance out the hip area, giving an hour-glass shape.

- Experiment with fabrics, textures and colour. You can choose fabrics that drape well and skim over the body instead of clinging. Accentuate curves with tailored jersey fabrics that pull in at the waist. Dark coloured bottoms will draw the eye to your top half, as will bold statement jewellery.

APPLE SHAPE

- Embrace empire waistlines that draw attention to the smallest part of the body (just below the bust) and flow over your middle. Or choose a classic shift dress that is tailored over the shoulder and skims across your middle with seams that give an illusion of shape. Shirt dresses that fit and flare will create shape at the waist even if you don't have it.

- Show off your slim legs with skirts or dresses that hit just above or below the knee. This can highlight your slim legs.

- Statement sleeves or details like ruffles, embellishments or a cold shoulder make a great focal point.

- Ruching and gathering can create the illusion of hourglass curves and hide a tummy if you want.

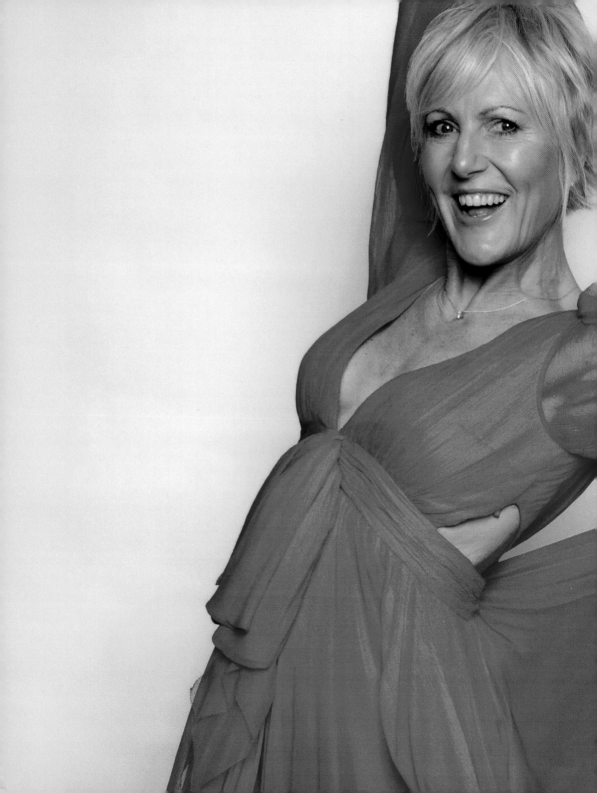

CHAPTER 12

CONGRATULATIONS

You've done it!

Please take time out to celebrate you and all you have achieved (if I could add sound and visual effects now, there would be a huge round of applause and a standing ovation).

BUT WHAT NEXT?

How can I help you maintain this new way of life beyond 90 days of creating new habits around mindset, nutrition and exercise?

A FEW POINTERS.

Stress management

You are probably not aware that stress has a big impact on weight management.

When stressed, the body releases a hormone called cortisol.

This can cause the following...

Increased Appetite: Cortisol can stimulate appetite, making you head to the fridge or snack cupboard for high-calorie comfort foods. It will send you to items high in sugar and fat, careering towards overeating and weight gain.

Fat Storage: Cortisol promotes the storage of fat, especially around the abdomen, which is the last thing we want after going through so much to shift it.

Muscle Loss: Elevated cortisol levels can lead to the breakdown of muscle tissue. As we know, muscle burns more calories than fat, so it reduces your body's ability to burn calories at rest. Less muscle mass means a slower metabolism.

Blood Sugar Imbalance: Cortisol can raise blood sugar levels. This triggers the release of insulin. Chronically high insulin levels can promote fat storage, particularly around the belly.

Reduced Physical Activity: Chronic stress, which often leads to elevated cortisol levels, can result in decreased physical activity and a sedentary lifestyle contributes to weight gain.

Poor Sleep: Stress and high cortisol levels can disrupt sleep patterns. Poor sleep is associated with weight gain and an increased risk of obesity.

You can help manage stress through relaxation techniques, exercise and a balanced lifestyle. This can help regulate cortisol levels and mitigate its impact on your weight.

Here are things I do to manage stress…

Keep a journal by my bed and note down anything stressful on my mind. I also try to make a list of things I need to do the next day. I definitely find this prevents me from waking in the night trying to remember them.

I then make a note of 3 things, large or small, that I am grateful for in my day. It takes your mind to a much more relaxed place, with positive thoughts before you sleep.

I avoid watching stressful things on TV before bed. I used to watch the News at 10 and of course it is rarely all good news. Without realising, the last thing I let enter my mind before I slept was something stressful. I now only watch it at 6pm.

I walk 20–30 mins, ideally among grass or trees and always without my headphones. The Japanese have "shinrin-yoku" or forest bathing as a health programme. Scientific studies have found that mindful walking for two hours in a forest reduced blood pressure, lowered cortisol and improved both concentration and memory. I have also been known to hug the odd, ancient tree!

CHOOSE HOLIDAYS THAT ARE HEALTHY

Holidays are often chances to slip back into bad habits of overindulgence or laziness.

Of course, it's all about balance. I try to find hotels or locations that enable me to enjoy some relaxing or sight-seeing, but also have great walks, a gym or a pool big enough to swim in.

If there are classes you can join in that's great, but if not you can find 15 mins in your room to do a HIIT workout.

I also tend not to book all-inclusive holidays.

As I mentioned in the section on preparation, it helped to remove temptation. I wouldn't eat a three-course meal every night at home, so why do I need it on holiday?

Finding a little local restaurant that you can walk to before choosing gorgeous fresh fish or chargrilled meat or vegetables is going to be far better for keeping on track with your new lifestyle.

Many organisations plan group trips and provide opportunities to explore new destinations with fellow travellers, if you want to meet new people with similar interests.

BRAVE THE COLD

As part of my 90 day challenge, alongside the diet and exercise programme, my personal trainer Joss added taking a 3 minute cold shower every morning to my list of things to do.

My first response was an internal shudder!

But, open to improving, I looked up the benefits to help get over the dread and there are many. It led me to look at more ways the cold can help. On top of the cold showers, I have tried ice baths (this is for the hardy) and I am now a big fan of cryotherapy chambers too. If I get to the British seaside, I will always brave the sea, although I am yet to do this in deepest winter – but I will!

So, what are the benefits?

Enhanced Muscle Recovery

We often see athletes and sportspeople in ice baths. This is because cold exposure accelerates muscle recovery after intense workouts or competitions. As I increased my level of exercise, I wanted to keep pushing myself and so I was keen to feel this benefit. Cold exposure also promotes faster recovery by helping remove waste products, such as lactic acid, from the muscles, helping reduce muscle fatigue and stiffness. Cold exposure helps mitigate the severity and duration of DOMS, accelerating recovery by reducing inflammation, promoting the repair of micro-tears in muscle tissue, reducing soreness and promoting faster healing. The cold temperature also constricts blood vessels, which may decrease swelling and tissue breakdown.

Boosted Metabolism and Weight Management

Research is ongoing into the difference in function characteristics between white fat and brown fat in the body. There is particular interest in how to activate brown fat with exposure to cold temperatures.

White fat's function is to store excess energy in the form of triglycerides. It serves as an energy reservoir for the body.

The primary function of brown fat is to generate heat in a process called thermogenesis. Brown fat cells contain a protein which allows them to produce heat. This process is crucial for maintaining body temperature.

The activation and presence of more brown fat versus white may have metabolic benefits, as it can burn calories to generate heat. This has led to interest in understanding and harnessing the potential of brown fat for supporting weight management and metabolic health, increasing calorie burning as the body works harder to generate heat

Improved Circulation

Quick and intense exposure to cold water causes blood vessels to constrict and then dilate when the body warms up. This process, known as vasoconstriction and vasodilation, improves blood circulation. This may help improve blood flow to various parts of the body, enhancing overall cardiovascular health.

Boosted Immune System

Regular exposure to cold water may stimulate the production of white blood cells, potentially supporting the immune system. This could enhance the body's ability to fight off infections.

Increased Respiratory Rate

Cold water exposure can lead to deeper and faster breathing, which may enhance lung capacity and oxygen intake. Certainly, breathing through the initial shock of the cold is a way of managing the body's urge to jump out of the icy water! This effect can be invigorating and beneficial for respiratory health, improving lung capacity over time.

Alleviation of Creaky, Painful Joints

With a family history of arthritis and joints that have stiffened with hormonal changes, this was a big plus for me. Cold exposure can have a pain-relieving effect which provides relief for joint pain or arthritis. It can temporarily numb the nerve endings, reducing pain perception and alleviating joint pain whilst improving mobility.

Increased Alertness and Energy

There's nothing like a cold shower to wake you up! Cold showers can stimulate the nervous system and lead to an increase in alertness and energy levels. The shock of cold water can induce a "cold stress response," which triggers the release of adrenaline and other neurotransmitters associated with wakefulness.

Improved Sleep Quality

Exposure to cold water can contribute to better sleep quality. The drop in body temperature after cold water immersion may help promote relaxation, regulate the sleep-wake cycle and promote restful sleep.

Mental Well Being

The icy cold shock of cold water can have an invigorating effect on the nervous system, prompting increased alertness and a boost in mood. It can trigger the release of endorphins, the body's natural feel-good hormones, leading to a sense of euphoria and reduced stress, alleviating symptoms of mild depression. I always felt more feeling, more energised and alert after cryotherapy sessions.

Improved Skin and Hair Health

Cold water can tighten pores, potentially reducing the risk of acne and promoting healthier skin. It may also contribute to shinier hair by closing hair cuticles and preventing moisture loss.

May Help Improve Appearance of Cellulite

Fat cells are sensitive to extreme cold and undergo self-destruction under freezing temperatures. When this happens fatty lumps and the bonds holding them together are eliminated, hence the claim that cold exposure supports cellulite reduction.

It's no secret that improved circulation can improve how your skin looks and reduce the appearance of cellulite.

If you're considering incorporating cold water or ice baths into your routine, it's advisable to consult with a healthcare professional or sports medicine expert to ensure it's appropriate for your own situation. If you have specific health concerns or conditions, it's always a good idea to seek personalised advice. There are considerations for safety and potential contraindications for individuals with certain medical conditions, such as cardiovascular issues.

If you are looking at cold water swimming, gradually acclimatise to colder temperatures to avoid risks such as hypothermia.

BE OPEN TO OPPORTUNITIES TO LEARN

As I write this, I have just finished climbing Kilimanjaro!

It wasn't on my bucket list for my 60th year, but when the opportunity came to join a team of 9 other intrepid women to raise money for The Prince's Trust, Women Supporting Women, I didn't hesitate.

I considered myself fit and love hiking so signed up without properly researching it. That was my first lesson! I had no idea what it really entailed and how hard it was, but I had committed, so there was no turning back. In our first planning call, I found out about the one-man tents, the altitude sickness and the vast kit list that would see me through 5 micro climates, from rainforest at the bottom, to arctic wastelands at the top of the mountain.

This was going to push me out of my comfort zone way more than I expected.

A LESSON IN HUMILITY

Before leaving for the expedition I went along for an altitude reaction assessment in order to gauge how my body would respond to the conditions at 5000m. I had a horrible shock. I reacted terribly, feeling as if I was being suffocated within 30 seconds with my heart pounding, lungs screaming for air and vision darkening. After initially feeling confident, I was suddenly plunged into feeling extremely inadequate. Ironically my fitness level played against me as I am used to using oxygen very efficiently. A sudden lack of it had an exaggerated effect. After this, I had to learn how to manage the fear of the unknown and the possibility that I might not make the top. I decided that all I could do was give it my all and try the best I could.

The good news was that I could use training to help my body adapt to altitude. I did this and fortunately it paid off.

BE GRATEFUL FOR WHAT YOU HAVE

Spending 7 nights in a one man tent with no running water, using a porta-loo and living with the smallest wardrobe of clothes, the little luxuries became really important. Friends lent me lots of fabulous kit including a top of the range sleeping bag, the warmest of quilted jackets, the perfect size rucksack and an insulated water bladder. I was given a few sumptuous miniature toiletries and invested in hand and feet warmers. The item that sticks with me is the loan of a spare toothbrush to clean my nails. 8 days living in volcanic mud and ash with only wet wipes to rely on, you never really felt clean. Oh, the joy of having clean nails, if only for a few minutes!

THE MIND CAN PUSH YOUR BODY FAR FURTHER THAN YOU THINK

We reached base camp after 6 days of climbing. The final push to reach the summit entailed 9 hours of stumbling up rocky boulders on a steep incline, leaving at 11.30pm so that all six of us were in darkness with just a head torch to light the way. With 25 mph winds and temperatures that dropped to -19 degrees, my body soon began to beg for it all to stop. My mind, however, found new realms of grit and determination. I called on deep reserves of motivation, thinking of family and those less fortunate. As I made it to the summit, waves of emotion overtook me; I felt a mix of exhilaration, pride and relief.

LASTLY, I LEARNED IT WAS OK NOT TO BE OK

I climbed with a wonderful group of kind, strong, successful women, some of whom I knew, most of whom I didn't. We were all there because we wanted to support disadvantaged young women.

We laughed a lot, but with the highs came lows and at some point, we all cried.

We lifted each other up whenever we noticed somebody needed it.

I deeply missed my home and family. We had no phone or internet signal so I couldn't tell them how much I missed them. I also missed familiar surroundings and my bed! Parts of the trip were far harder than I could ever have dreamed of.

It was strangely liberating to not put on a brave face with people I had never met before. Somehow being stripped bare of normal expectations brought emotions much closer to the surface. I realised that it was ok not to be ok.

Now, I am not suggesting to anyone that they rush off and climb Kilimanjaro. But do be open to new experiences, you will learn something about yourself. Of that you can be sure.

SET YOURSELF NEW GOALS

This is an important one. For example, I absolutely love dancing! I have had Salsa and Jive lessons and bought new tap shoes during lockdown to keep myself entertained. I am sharing with you now that my next goal is to be on Strictly Come Dancing! I am manifesting it, so it has to happen!

I am creating my vision board. The outfits, the glitter ball, picturing which movie I will cover and my Halloween Week special look. The only question is which male dancer do I pick? I will leave you with that thought. I just hope you vote for me when I am on!

SO, WHAT'S NEXT FOR YOU?

We have reached the end, but in reality, it is just the end of the beginning. This is not the end of your journey because that is one that will only grow more exciting as you keep learning and opening up to new experiences.

In a world often fixated on youth, there's a remarkable treasure hidden in celebrating the course of our lives so far, no matter our age.

AND WHAT'S NEXT FOR ME?

I want to keep learning. The more I read and learn about the impact of diet, exercise and positive thinking for the body and mind, the more I realise we can do so many things to help ourselves. I see so much potential.

I decided it was time to explore why life truly begins at 60 and the myriad ways this stage of life can be the most fulfilling and transformative of all.

I am going to make the most of feeling invincible not invisible.